The author has worked for 45 years in the care and nursing profession, principally with people who have learning disabilities. He was a Ward Manager and Home Manager for 30 years, developing pioneering community services for people with learning disabilities and complex emotional needs. Currently, he is the Positive Behavioural Support Manager and a Quality Auditor for Milestones Trust, a leading provider of social care services in Bristol and its surrounding area. He also is an Associate Lecturer at the University of the West of England.

I would like to dedicate this book to all the service users and colleagues that I have met and worked with over the last 45 years and who have provided me with such inspiration throughout my career.

Alan Nuttall

CARING FOR THE CARERS

A Guide to Help Paid Carers for People with
Learning Disabilities

AUSTIN MACAULEY PUBLISHERS™

LONDON • CAMBRIDGE • NEW YORK • SHARJAH

A CIP catalogue record for this title is available from the British Library.

ISBN 9781787101043 (Paperback)
ISBN 9781528952699 (ePub e-book)

www.austinmacauley.com

First Published (2019)
Austin Macauley Publishers Ltd
25 Canada Square
Canary Wharf
London
E14 5LQ

I would like to acknowledge the support of my wife, Paulette; my children, Kathryn, Hannah, Philip and Sophie, particularly Sophie for proofreading before submission; and the support of close colleagues who encouraged me and read my work, feeding back that it wasn't complete rubbish.

Introduction

This book concerns itself with the causes of stress for paid carers who work with people with learning disabilities in a variety of settings ranging from treatment centres and specialised medium secure hospitals to residential care homes and supported living projects. It seeks to delineate approaches and strategies that are helpful to alleviate that stress.

As is appropriate, research concerning those who have intellectual disabilities focuses on their needs. However, the existence of very specific stressors relating to members of this client group and the impact on those who support them has been recognised for over twenty years, having been described by Sherrard in 1989 and Emerson et al in 1995.

There is a growing body of academic literature relating to this subject. Unfortunately, access to the valuable findings emanating from this research is not readily available to carers who work in this field.

No longer are carers expected to respond to, for instance, the distress caused by the death of people they support or the anxiety attendant on exposure to aggressive assaults in a stoical, emotionally detached manner.

Nevertheless, the complexities and range of stressors are still not fully appreciated by care workers and their supervisors; helpful approaches tend to be relatively unsophisticated and applied inconsistently. It is imperative that this issue is addressed principally to ensure the welfare of carers.

However, there are other factors which should be noted: employers have a legal duty under Health and Safety legislation to do all they can to protect the welfare of their workforces and that includes issues relating to emotional and psychological distress. They also have a moral duty to fulfil this requirement, although pragmatically actions that mitigate the impact of distress favour employers also, by reducing the incidence of absenteeism which is an inevitable consequence of job strain. Finally, and most importantly, carers who are stressed and demoralised are less likely to have positive interactions with service users, become apathetic and indifferent, with a weakening of values and moral sense This is an insidious process that can culminate in a 'corruption of care' described by Patterson and others (2011) and, as long ago as 1993, by Wardhaugh and Wilding.

In writing this book I have drawn on the literature produced over the last five years which is relevant to this subject. However, it would be extremely perverse of me to ignore what I have learned experientially during that period; for twenty years I have substantially been engaged in developing new, community-based services for people with learning disabilities who also have poor mental health, autism or become easily distressed and express their anger with aggression or other challenges to services. The process of creating, nurturing and managing staff teams throughout this period has inevitably exposed me to situations of staff distress and tension for which I have had to find solutions. Therefore, I have included perspectives arising from those experiences when they seem pertinent. When I have written about experiences of people that I have known, whether service user, staff or relative – I have changed names to preserve confidentiality.

A few words on terminology: people who support clients who have learning disabilities have many different job names, including health care assistant (HCA), support worker and personal assistant (PA). Often terms reflect the type or degree of support that is required so an HCA is more likely to be involved with a high degree of intimate care, sometimes in a more clinical setting whilst the role of a PA might be more to provide social care in a supported living environment. I have opted generally to use the term 'carer' as a short hand which encompasses all those different roles, even if some don't entail the more traditional aspects of 'care'.

Similarly, people with learning disabilities who have received services in a variety of contexts have been called inmates, patients, clients, tenants and service users, depending on the ethos of the time or their legal status. I have tended to use the term 'service user' throughout the book because, although unwieldy, it covers a whole range of environments that people may live in such as hospitals, care homes, supported living projects.

Also, I have settled for using the term 'learning disabilities', throughout the book, which should be regarded by readers as synonymous with all the other current descriptions of this client group, such as 'intellectual disabilities', 'learning difficulties' and 'developmental disabilities'. Language within this field quickly becomes archaic and derogatory, as attested by our negative attitudes to terms like 'mental retardation', 'mental subnormality' and 'mental handicap' which have commonly been used during the last three decades. No doubt 'learning disabilities' will suffer this fate ultimately, but for now it is regarded as respectful form of description by both practitioners and the academic community.

Chapter 1
What's the Problem?
What Exactly Are the Stressors Which Impinge
on the Health and Well-Being of Carers?

During the previous thirty years, there have been many
positive changes in the way that people with learning
disabilities are regarded and supported. When I first started
nurse training at Stoke Park Hospital in 1976, with the
intention of qualifying as nurse for, incredibly, the mentally
subnormal, great numbers of people with learning disabilities
still lived in large institutions often situated in remote areas
distant from towns and cities. Stoke Park Hospital, half a
mile's distance from the nearest easterly suburbs of Bristol,
accommodated over 500 women, men and children in 'wards'
populated by numbers ranging from 16 to 30 'patients', as
everyone including those who lived there termed the hospital
residents.

The majority of the Stoke Park Hospital population was
female or children, a relic of the gender segregation that was
imposed on the learning-disabled population who were
housed in the 'colonies' that were created in the early part of
the twentieth century. This appertained locally until the
beginning of the 1970s when some reciprocal integration took
place, usually against the wishes of service users, between
Stoke Park and its neighbour Purdown Hospital, which until
then had catered for an exclusively male population.

The perimeter of Bristol was studded with six other
institutions devoted to the accommodation of people with
learning disabilities which had populations ranging from 250
to 500. Even during the latter decades of the twentieth

century, children were being admitted to long term care at Stoke Park and its sister hospitals.

Both residents and staff testify to terrible abuses inflicted on people living in virtually unregulated, unmonitored and unvisited environments, included predatory sexual abuse by older, stronger male residents of adolescent boys transferred to male only institutions and beatings inflicted on 'patients' by staff.

Also, hospital residents were assailed by a multitude of less obvious abuses and deprivations. Although much improved compared to what had been the case even the previous decade, levels of staff support were unbelievably low. For example, it was usual for a group of eighteen to twenty incontinent, immobile, profoundly physically and mentally disabled adults who required all possible help with personal care to be cared for by only three or four members of staff.

If even the most unambitious social activity was contemplated, it had to take place in large numbers. I recollect an instance when I, during my second student nurse placement, supervised a group of twelve middle aged ladies with mild to moderate learning disabilities when we went for a walk in the surrounding countryside.

On another occasion, a care worker and I accompanied eight far less able ladies, who would now be termed as challenging, whilst they attended a disco at a neighbouring long stay hospital. Unsurprisingly, this situation culminated with me having to impose an improvised form of restraint on a lady who had hit several other service users for twenty minutes whilst I awaited the arrival of our transport.

Choice regarding even the most basic activities of living was virtually non-existent. Food was cooked in a large central kitchen with no consultation with residents about what they would like to eat or variation of times when meals took place.

Sleeping areas on wards consisted of open dormitories accommodating ten to twenty people with little space between beds and minimal individual storage facilities. No one who lived in these circumstances had the facility to lock away personal possessions, which were usually very few in number. It was usual for clothes to be kept in a central store cupboard; sometimes items were named, often not, leading to staff allocating 'communal' underwear to residents based on size and need.

The general environment was really unpleasant. Often wards smelled of faeces and urine. I remember vividly a cockroach the size of one of my fingers scuttling out of a service user's bedding whilst I was helping her to get up.

The washing of clothes was done at a large laundry not located on the hospital site which catered for the needs of several residential institutions. As a consequence, there was plenty of scope for the loss of precious and cherished personal items.

Frequently, hospital residents had conditions such as autism or epilepsy, concerning which the staff had little knowledge and understanding, or had mental health issues which were undiagnosed or treated inadequately. There was hardly any awareness of the long-term effects on people's mental state, self-esteem and levels of motivation due to living in institutions where levels of independence, privacy, individuality and choice were so circumscribed.

Documentation about the needs and activities of 'patients' was minimal; many times, I saw a whole decade of a person's life summed up in a dozen totally unconnected, sometimes derogatory entries written on a single sheet of A4 paper. It was also possible to read antiquated and pejorative terminology in people's notes categorising them as 'idiots', 'morons' or 'imbeciles'.

Even at the height of the institutional model of care, the majority of people with a learning disability did not live in long stay hospitals. Nevertheless, significantly large numbers did, particularly if they had profound impairments or complex emotional needs. The hospital system stands as compelling testimony to the devalued and discriminatory attitudes that were generally afforded to those who had disabilities.

Nowadays, the way that people with intellectual disabilities are supported is by no means perfect – the exposure of care delivered at Winterbourne View provides extreme but telling evidence that this is so – however, there have been many improvements.

Generally, people live, at the worst, in care homes which are situated in local communities instead of being geographically remote and where the principles of person-centred support are reasonably well established. Increasingly, people with learning disabilities live in 'supported living' projects where support is closely matched to an individual's assessed needs.

Instead of losing touch with their disabled relatives, family members are encouraged to be intimately involved in care and support. This is in stark contrast to what was prevalent in the era of long stay institutions when even parents were discouraged from visiting their learning-disabled children. Sometimes access was limited to days stipulated by the hospital administrators rather than those convenient for family members.

Those who have a learning disability are still more likely to have a mental illness or be subjected to many different abuses. They still run the risk of being effectively incarcerated in secure hospitals due to aggressive behaviour or persistent, but minor, offences. However, at least there is now a body of knowledge and research which can inform carers and supporters how to support learning disabled people who do have psychiatric disorders. There is an increasing understanding of risk factors for abuse and how to recognise its presentation in vulnerable people who cannot readily communicate, backed by legal sanctions around safeguarding and inspection requirements.

The greater respect which is afforded to people with intellectual disabilities is reflected in the terminology that is now prevalent concerning their status: no longer are they referred to as 'patients', 'high grades' and 'low grades' (the latter, incidentally a term commonly used by hospital residents, as an insult towards their compatriots). Instead people with disabilities are given designations like 'service user', 'client' or 'tenant', all indicative of a more valued place in the community.

One of the most telling changes over the last 30 years is that the majority of people with learning disabilities are brought up in their own families and generally live in the same communities and neighbourhoods as the rest of the population using the same facilities and services as everyone else.

I felt that it was important to at least allude briefly to the experiences that patients, residents, service users, clients and tenants (to use the various forms of nomenclature applied to people with learning disabilities since the 1970s) in part to provide a salutary reminder of the difficulties faced by one of society's most disadvantaged sectors which, notwithstanding recent positive developments, can easily re-emerge. It is well to remember that however distressed carers might become, the lives of service users contain a much greater risk of being exposed to adverse and damaging events and interactions.

Nevertheless, I make no apology for focussing on the support needs of carers, a group of people who also have been neglected over the years. Moreover, the lives and experiences of staff members and service users are intimately linked; often paid carers are the most significant people involved in the lives of those who have disabilities. Stress factors can at the very least reduce the quality of interactions between the former and the latter and become a predicator for extremely abusive practices.

So, why does a book need to be written on this subject? After all, carers, nurses, personal assistants have all chosen their particular career willingly and have done so with an appreciation of the stressors that they will encounter, haven't they? And are those stressors any worse than those met by carers who support other dependent groups or any workers in completely different fields such as retail, education or business?

Certainly, an understanding of the pressures felt by carers for people with learning disabilities was acknowledged even thirty years ago by Sharrard (1989).

Awareness amongst care staff of the causes of stress and its effects was very limited though. For example, the approach that was commonplace in the long stay hospitals was that carers should be stoical, unemotional or even callous about matters such as the death of residents. When the death of Brian occurred during my first hospital placement, a lad who could not walk, speak, recognise others, feed or dress himself, those few sensitive souls who cried at his passing were derided by their tougher colleagues who regarded the child's death as a welcome relief for everyone, including, incidentally, Brian himself. Absolutely no one reflected on the long-term effects of processing the emotional impact of such deaths, which were by no means uncommon.

Nevertheless, when service users die, the people who have supported them often for many years are bound to be affected, but also perhaps confused with regard to what their response should be. Carers are encouraged to maintain a certain detachment from service users and not become emotionally involved. They should never lose sight of the fact that they are not friends but paid supporters who must focus all their energies in helping those that they support develop relationships and interests within the local community, consistent with modern philosophy as encapsulated in O'Brien's five accomplishments.

However, this is an aim which is often difficult to achieve, particularly if someone has a profound disability or a condition like autism, which prevents him or her readily making friends, or have lost contact with family due to a life time in long term care. Almost inevitably, people with learning disabilities who are disadvantaged in the ways I have intimated come to regard their carers as the most important people in their lives, and the latter reciprocate, becoming attached to people who have so few significant friendships and contacts.

The response to the death of someone with a disability whom you have supported for many years is likely to be similar to that experienced by the workforce in the following example:

A few years ago, Donald, a middle-aged man with a moderate learning disability, who charmed everyone with his humour and eccentric habits, died unexpectedly after a short illness. He had lived in a community home that I managed for five years, after residing in a hospital since he was a child. The staff who had supported Donald were traumatised and distraught; they ranged from being tearful, argumentative, angry or flinging themselves into activities such as clearing his room. When his father initially stated his wish for Donald to have a quiet funeral, they were up in arms at this suggestion, wanting him to have a funeral to which everyone who knew him would be invited as a celebration of his short life.

Of course, people die in all sorts of walks of life, especially in care settings. However, the sophisticated but ambiguous approach that supporters of people with learning disabilities are expected to adopt causes tensions. Carers partake in so many intimate areas of someone's life but not assume the status of friendship, and so a particularly nuanced form of support is required, especially if carers blame themselves for the causes of death.

Probably the most well researched source of stress for carers is the field of 'challenging behaviour' an area which in the past was disregarded as no one acknowledged the impact of aggression perpetrated by service users on staff, who were encouraged to simply 'get on with it' should they have had the misfortune to be attacked.

However, challenges are not confined to instances of physical aggression such as being kicked, punched, scratched, pinched, or hit by objects. Here are some examples of antisocial, disruptive or distressing behaviour that I have encountered during my career and have also been described in academic articles:

Spitting; faecal smearing or urinating in inappropriate locations; being sworn at; having hurtful things said to you (the most distressing comment that I have heard uttered by a service user to a colleague is 'I hope your baby dies'); service users harming themselves by hitting their heads, gouging their eyes, biting or scratching themselves, attacking fellow residents, stripping off in public places, repetitive questioning, screaming and shouting.

The type of emotional responses to such behaviours are also well documented and include feelings of anger, disgust, fear, guilt (from failing to support service users adequately), remorse (for having negative feelings towards clients), sense of helplessness and despair (Emerson et al 1995).

It is obvious that those staff members that support people with learning disabilities who challenge are not, apart from extremely exceptional circumstances, placed in situations of life-threatening danger, unlike members of the armed forces and the police. Also, there is great understanding nowadays that problematic and dysfunctional behaviours are likely to be a form of communication that we have a professional and moral duty to try our utmost to understand. Similarly, carers are aware of the many long-term factors which might lead to people with learning disabilities becoming distressed such as long-term institutionalisation, subjection to abuse, psychiatric disorders and autism, all of which they are more likely to experience than any other section of the population.

Notwithstanding the emotions such as fear, anger or disgust, felt by carers often 'in the heat of the moment', are very powerful and must cause tremendous turmoil in people who aspire to have a calm caring approach to those that they support. On a daily basis, staff members have to maintain a subtle balance between being non-confrontational, supportive and assertive when dealing with people who are potentially aggressive, requiring a conscious mastery of body language, facial expression, and tone, pitch and volume of voice which are completely unnatural and difficult to achieve when one is frightened, perplexed or anxious due to problematical behaviour. After aggressive incidents, carers may be self-recriminatory because they think they have failed the people that they support or feel emotionally and physically drained or embarrassed.

Besides, those feelings can contribute to care staff attributing the causes of behaviour to negative reasons that are assumed to be controllable by service users displaying challenging behaviour, leading to them to develop resentful and condemnatory attitudes. Obviously, this process with its inevitable conclusion of some degree of stigmatisation will impact primarily on those people who express their distress through dysfunctional actions. Nevertheless, attributions which are unhelpful and unconstructive and promote the practice of blaming disabled individuals for their actions affect the well-being of carers, because they distract them from developing a true understanding of the problematic behaviours, what their functions are, and how they could be addressed in a supportive manner, and so lead to the perpetuation of the very behaviours that have caused the initial negative response.

The phenomenon of self-injurious behaviour, manifesting, for example, as individuals biting, pinching, gouging, cutting or hitting themselves, occurs in approximately 17% of the learning-disabled population, and, by definition, impacts on those who display such traits. Nevertheless, research relating to the emotional effect of self-harm on carers indicates that they can experience strong feelings of sadness, despair and guilt, sometimes degenerating into apathy and indifference due to their inability to fully understand or ameliorate such apparently inexplicable and bizarre behaviours.

Indeed, the causes and functions of self-injurious behaviour can be diverse and vary between individuals: one person may be seeking to ward off demands and attention from others whilst another may be attempting to seek gratification of his or her needs. It may be an expression of distress which is a response to a very specific stressor such as pain or to an entire panoply of frustrations, immediate or otherwise or else a form of self-stimulation to raise levels of stimulation. The presence of a sensory deficit may contribute to the likelihood of someone harming themselves. It may be a form of self-punishment or specifically a consequence of self-loathing caused by sexual abuse. There is an association with conditions such as autism and the extremely limited communication abilities linked to profound intellectual disability. Self-injurious behaviour may be specifically related to rare but significant illnesses, such as Lesch-Nyhan and Prader-Willi Syndromes. The interplay between such factors may be complex and historical, knowledge of which is not easily attained and understood by carers.

Understanding of the causes of challenging behaviour and models of support such as Positive Behavioural Support is frequently the norm within the work force, knowledge which is both beneficial to service users and heartening for staff who have access to proactive strategies, in itself a form of coping strategy. Nevertheless, challenges may endure for many years, progress in moderating them and nurturing development can be agonisingly slow resulting in feelings of burnout and diminished job satisfaction.

Carers are drawn from very diverse origins, and sometimes are subjected to racial abuse. Although this occurs in all walks of life, it is an issue that cannot always be readily addressed to the complete satisfaction of the member of staff being abused. This is due to the difficulty in imposing sanctions in a care setting; the limited means that disabled individuals may have to learn from debriefing about the inappropriateness of racist comments; and the perception as a mitigating factor that racial abusers who have learning disabilities may have had extremely poor role models either in their family or the long stay institutions that they lived in during less enlightened eras.

Paid supporters of people with learning disabilities are rightly urged to assess and manage risk for their clients, rather than adopt a risk adverse attitude which militates against service users' aspirations to live a full and interesting life. Pursuing such a course can be fraught with tension though, since there may be consequences that can be hard for staff to manage however comprehensive the relevant risk assessments. Carers may have to deal with situations which cause them anxiety, fear or embarrassment, such as when service users accost or touch members of the public inappropriately, take off their clothes, relieve themselves in public or attempt to run off from those who are accompanying them.

There are other aspects inherent in the care of people with learning disabilities which can cause tension for their supporters. Many people with profound disabilities cannot communicate verbally to any significant degree and may appear to be totally unaware of their surroundings or the interactions of other people. A possible outcome might be that their personal assistants will find such a disproportionately unequal relationship unfulfilling and ultimately dispiriting. Relationships like these occur with other groups of people such as infant children and the elderly. However, parents know that even the youngest baby will develop an awareness of others within few weeks, whilst relationships with senior citizens who have dementia are strengthened and enriched through knowledge of their former valued roles, achievements and contributions to society. Someone with a profound intellectual impairment does not hold out the prospect of any development within months or even years or have a compensatory back story which enhances the sense of worth that others may have for him or her.

A similar phenomenon may occur with regard to relationships with people who have autism and so find it difficult to interact with others or even withdraw into their own circumscribed world displaying little empathy and understanding of other people's needs and emotions. As with those with profound disabilities, the reaction over a course of years might be a sense of tedium and despair in supporting people who appear to give back so little.

The need for support with incontinence or personal hygiene is not exclusive to the learning-disabled client group but is more likely to be accompanied by dysfunctional or antisocial behaviours. Also, people with learning disabilities may be perceived as having an inability to interact meaningfully or develop significantly and take an active role in the community. Dealing with the bodily functions of adults in particular is a difficult task requiring a very positive and understanding outlook which is hard to sustain over a lengthy period of time without mitigating factors such as the prospect of development.

Another possible source of stress for carers is the fluctuating nature of how others have perceived their role through the years. Many years ago, the function of staff was to provide custodial care which aimed to fulfil basic physical needs but ignored emotional and social wants. As the move towards community care progressed, the expectation was that staff help service users attain the whole gamut of experiences, even though they may be ill-equipped to do so due to lack of social skills and an extensive community network. Nevertheless, staff members were expected to help those people who lived secluded lives in hospitals rapidly. Carers who gave some of their own personal time to their role were seen as better than those who simply did their allocated hours.

In recent years the view has predominated that carers should adopt an enabling role, encouraging service users to become independent and nurturing relationships while maintaining a certain distance and discouraging the notion that carers are friends with their clientele. Role ambiguity has been identified by Hatton et al (1999) as a cause of job strain particularly amongst younger, less well-trained members of staff.

In reality the role of carers is much more complex and multifaceted than any of the above accounts. It has evolved to being one which is facilitative rather than protective. However, circumstances arise in which carers may need to exert influence to ensure the safety of the people that they support or may entail a more traditional caring approach due to the needs of very severely disabled individuals. Also, it is not always possible to avoid blurring the lines between work and home life. As part of their job, personal assistants have access to a lot of intimate information concerning people to whom they provide a service and it seems really discordant not to disclose at least some details about one's personal life. Also, it is difficult to avoid generating emotional attachments to clients when you work so closely with them, as sometimes it is hard to forget your home life whilst supporting people in their own homes when you are experiencing personal distress.

People who have been employed for many years may be stigmatised because of the assumption by senior managers that those who participated formerly in outdated models of care are inevitably incapable of adaption and unable to embrace modern approaches. Conversely, a carer who has been appointed who seemingly fits the criteria set by senior managers with regard to person centeredness etc may endure stress because of an overestimation of abilities and a failure to appreciate the impact of a lack of experience in coping with adverse situations.

Carers are particularly susceptible to criticism from other professionals who may visit care homes to offer advice, sometimes in a highly judgemental way without having any great understanding of the stresses that they are subjected to. Support workers are often drawn from many different backgrounds, find it difficult to refute or accept criticism from better educated and apparently more articulated external colleagues and may resent the intervention of people who have limited appreciation of their work constraints.

There may be a dissonance between the values and attitudes of the parent organisation and members of the work force who deliver direct support. A care provider may be a profit making company whose primary objective of maximised returns may lead to a perceived or actual diminution in resources devoted to the client group, such as a reduction in staff/client ratios causing carers to be disaffected on behalf of their service users whose lives become more circumscribed and less person orientated due that reduction.

It seems anomalous that the culture, as expressed through the actions and approaches of senior managers, of an organisation that ostensibly aspires to provide person centred services in a caring facilitate manner can become quite aggressive and authoritarian, leading to uncertainty and a lowering of morale due to the disparity between the humanistic approaches of carers and the demands made by managers. This process may result from the inherent personalities of the people involved or be a consequence of financial constraints or the negative impact of external inspection and audit. A 'top down' approach to management can have the effect of employees feeling disempowered, demotivated and distressed because their views and experience are not valued, and they are given few opportunities to use their initiative and demonstrate creativity. Hatton et al (1999) identified that organisational characteristics were just as significant as a cause of job strain as those relating to service users and staff. The same writers identify that bureaucracy and lack of support for staff leads to the development of highly emotional and unhelpful 'wishful' thinking styles of coping instead of more useful problem-solving approaches.

External professionals comprise one group of staff with whom care workers may find it difficult to maintain a sense of solidarity and common purpose, because the former do not have to work unsocial hours. Similarly, carers may feel estranged from their organisation's senior managers or administrative personnel for the same reason and the perception that members of these groups have little understanding of the problems direct care workers encounter.

When service users attend hospital appointments or admitted for treatment as in-patients, they are sometimes met with a complete lack of understanding from doctors and nurses of those institutions, especially if they have complex emotional needs or a severe communication deficit. The burden falls on support staff to act as a mediator and advocate for their clients and to be a guide in matters of best interests and mental capacity, roles fraught with complexity and a heightened sense of responsibility. It has been observed by (reference) that general hospital staff frequently have significantly negative attitudes towards people with learning disabilities which have to be countered and overcome by direct carers who are supporting their clients in these clinical contexts.

One of the more onerous aspects of working life that residential and supported living staff experience is the extreme unsociability of the hours that they work. They may be rostered to fulfil early, late and night shifts over a relatively short period of time with an inevitable detrimental effect on sleep patterns and routine. Of course, there is an obligation to be on duty during times when most of the working population are on holiday, such as during the Christmas and New Year period. Most carers are obliged to work regularly on weekends also. Such work patterns affect people's ability to lead a normal social life, pursue hobbies and interests and participate fully in family life. They may be further exacerbated by the requirement to do 'sleep-ins', the provision of cover overnight at the disabled person's home, for a fairly small payment, in excess of core hours. 'Sleep-ins' can affect staff by taking them away from their families for several nights a week, adding to levels of fatigue because of the need to provide support during the night even though one might be working in the morning and generally contributing to the sense of dislocation from conventional life.

Often carers find it difficult to sleep well in the workplace whether they are disturbed by clients or not, due to the inability to wind down after an evening supporting service users and then trying to settle down immediately to sleep without a period of transition away from the workplace. Simply sleeping in an environment which is different to home can be disruptive and lead to broken sleep and consequent fatigue during the following day.

'Sleeping-in' is one example of the practice of 'lone working' which carers increasingly have to endure. Night work or support for someone who lives by him or herself may also entail long periods of working by oneself. Inevitably, people can feel vulnerable and apprehensive in these circumstances because of the fear of intruders, the extra tension attendant on coping with problematic behaviour by oneself and the exponential increase in stress due to working long periods of unsocial hours in isolation.

Parents and relatives of those who have a learning disability frequently find it difficult when their family members leave home to commence living in a residential or supported living service. Having devoted many years to caring for their children themselves often entailing many sacrifices, parents especially may feel several emotions: a sense of loss or even grief because their child is no longer the focus of their life, elation due to a new found sense of freedom and diminished responsibility, guilt for having such apparently self-centred thoughts and also for no longer fulfilling their caring role, and resentment towards carers for apparently usurping many aspects of their parental duties.

There may be a great disparity between the views each party may have regarding how someone with a learning disability should be supported; often family members adopt a more protective approach whilst paid personal assistants may be more inclined to encourage their clients to take risks and lead a more independent life. This potential dichotomy is a potent source of dispute and conflict which can affect both parties. It is entirely understandable that parents who have devotedly raised their disabled children, overcoming many difficulties adopt the view that their knowledge of those children cannot be bettered, and they inevitably know what is best for their offspring. However sensitive and understanding carers are, it is difficult for them to interact with families who vociferously express views of this nature. Sometimes the ideas concerning care that parents assert are at variance with how their children wish to live their lives. For instance, they may not agree with them going out unescorted or have objections to them forming sexual relationships causing conflicts in which carers consider themselves bound to support and advocate for the service user, leading to acrimonious and stressful disputes.

Parents also may insist that their disabled children follow cultural practices such as dietary restrictions or observing forms of worship which may conflict with the wishes of the individual and appear to be an imposition which is discordant with the concept of person-centred support.

Also, although family members may have an excellent knowledge of their relative's history and personal characteristics, they may not have detailed understanding of medical conditions that might be present, such as autism, Fragile X, epilepsy or schizophrenia, all of which learning disabled are more likely to have compared to the general population. Carers may have more expertise regarding those sorts of disorders and a different view as to their effect on behaviour, personality and well-being, perhaps resulting in disputes with parents or siblings who have a less sophisticated level of comprehension. Obviously, it might also be the case that parents have a really detailed knowledge of the conditions that their children have, and tension is cause by the deficiency in understanding displayed by paid carers.

The entire area of risk management is fraught with difficulty for paid staff members who are caught between the imperative to encourage independence and risk taking whilst guarding against circumstances which might lead to a service user becoming vulnerable to danger or abuse. Carers perpetually run the risk of being criticised for being risk averse or for displaying negligence and failing to safeguard the people that they are responsible for.

Sometimes clients have pressing health care needs or issues of safety which means that their capacity to make decisions has to be assessed and a decision has to be made as to whether to pursue a course of action and support which that person might resist but is deemed to be necessary in his or her 'best interests'.

The Mental Capacity Act, its accompanying code of practice and Deprivation of Liberty safeguards have been extremely progressive and helpful developments which guide staff through the process of balancing the rights of service users to make their own decisions with the need for supporters to intervene when there are compelling reasons to do so. Also, these instruments confer on carers and others the obligations to involve family members, Independent Mental Capacity Assessors, other professionals, Deprivation of Liberty Assessors and anyone else who is significant. Nevertheless in these circumstances, it is usually paid carers, particularly home and project managers, who initiate this process, which can be fraught with potential anguish as decisions may be made which impose actions or sanctions that reassure carers that they have fulfilled their 'duty of care', but are seemingly divergent from the current philosophical and ethical approach.

An example of this is the use, in extreme circumstances, of restraint procedures with service users who have severe intellectual deficits and potentially serious illnesses in order to facilitate venepuncture or other clinical investigations. Although carers, who inevitably are supporters, participants or observers of such procedures, may understand very well that such actions are very necessary to ensure effective diagnosis and treatment of perhaps life threatening illnesses about which the service users has no comprehension at all, the use of such extremely restrictive strategies and the distress that they elicit in the client can be extremely upsetting for them.

It is an expectation in all caring fields that employees demonstrate a commitment to the principles of equality and diversity. In practice this may entail supporting clients in activities and duties which are at variance with carers' deeply held moral beliefs. For instance, a vegetarian may have to prepare a meal for a service user which entails cooking meat, or someone from one particular religious persuasion may be required to help a client to worship at a church of a completely different denomination. Carers may have to turn a blind eye to pornographic materials or support someone who engages in alternative sexual practices which they might consider highly offensive or immoral even though they are legal. Sometimes their job might entail supporting a client who has offended against the law in ways that potentially give rise to strong emotions, such as in the case of sex offenders, causing staff extreme tension and anguish as they strive to preserve a non-judgemental and professional approach (Sandhu and others 2012).

People with learning disabilities are probably more likely than anyone else from the general community to be victims of abuse. Maltreatment can be perpetrated by fellow service users, paid carers, friends or family members and can take the form of physical or sexual assault, emotional cruelty, bullying or intimidation. Ill treatment may entail financial exploitation, neglect or denial of various basic rights.

Carers take a high proportion of the burden and stress consequent to dealing with mistreatment of their client group. Often staff members are the first people to become aware of abuse; they may be distressed themselves in encountering upsetting situations or have highly conflicting emotions if the perpetrator is a close colleague or a member of the service user's family. They may feel guilty for a perceived failing on their own part for allowing abuse to have taken or at the very least failing to anticipate it. Victims may not wish to have what they have disclosed shared with the authorities which may cause carers anguish due to the tension between the responsibility they bear to report safeguarding incidents and their wish to retain the trust of clients and preserve their confidentiality. Staff may be blamed and disciplined by their parent organisation for delays in following policies and reporting abusive situations; their actions may be scrutinised and denigrated by external professionals at safeguarding review meetings.

There is one faction of staff who are particularly prone to stress, namely the one comprising home and project managers. As well as bearing the ultimate responsibility for a service and being very conscious that they would be held accountable for any deficits in care and support, care managers suffer from a variety of other stressors. Often the variety of roles that they are expected to fill are inherently ambiguous and conflicting frequently entail providing direct care and support to service users as well as being a manager.

Home and project managers usually have to address the concerns raised by stakeholders other than the obvious ones of the staff team and the client group. They have to deal with relatives, external professionals, maintenance staff, CQC inspectors and organisational personnel, many of whom have little appreciation of the demands of managing a service for people with learning disabilities and are expected to be patient and helpful in all circumstances. During a period 'on duty', a manager may be required to adopt a variety of approaches, from being an assertive leader who is highly directive, to adopting a more facilitative, enabling approach or being a mentor, counsellor or teacher. He or she may have to manage staff conflict or indiscipline and critical situations relating to clients' health, safety or safeguarding whilst maintaining a positive and constructive long-term view of the service.

Home and project managers may develop close relationships with team members based on a shared experience of adversity, emotional response to difficulties or indeed through a sense of achievement as service users are supported to develop and achieve a more fulfilled lifestyle. They may come to regard their teams as their main source of emotional support. However, developing such relationships is perilous because there may be occasions when a manager has to address concerns raised by the actions of team members relating to areas such as prolonged absence due to illness, conflicts been individuals or poor performance, which militate against having a close relationship within junior staff and impair the manager's support network.

Sometimes, more senior managers may have never have been a residential home or supported living project manager and have a limited appreciation or understanding of either the work load or the emotional impact of these roles; the supervision that they give may be more functional, administrative or finance driven and insensitive to what might be regarded as the 'softer' demands on home and project managers.

Home and project managers often feel that they are 'on duty' for twenty-four hours every single day. Team members sometimes ring them for advice or to inform them about crisis situations and controversial incidents in the evenings, weekends, even the middle of the night. These occurrences can cause family tensions and the perception that one is never able to escape the stresses of work.

Increasingly, managers feel highly scrutinised by a plethora of internal and external monitoring agencies, including CQC, organisational audit processes, environmental health inspectors, commissioners and service purchasers. They frequently feel the need to prioritise updating documentation or meeting demands for information to protect themselves from criticism, whilst being aware that this approach may appear to contradict the principle of being person centred and always putting the needs of service users first.

As has been noted above, sometimes service users need to be the focus of mental capacity assessments and 'best interests' discussions as a response to serious health care and safety concerns, particularly if their learning disability is severe or they have complex emotional or psychiatric needs. The responsibility for initiating this process, resolving any disputes between people who are significant to the service user and negotiating what might be a restrictive course of action is shouldered by the home or project manager. This process can be a tremendous burden for that manager as she professionally and objectively tries to resolve any conflicts, including difference of views amongst members of the staff team, and to ensure that 'duty of care' obligations are fulfilled and essential treatment is delivered whilst being emotionally affected herself by contemplating using restrictive practices. Although decisions taken may be shared, it is possible that a home/project manager will have a heightened sense of accountability having been involved throughout in the process.

Nowadays, although they may be very able and have received training to perform this difficult amalgam of duties and functions, managers that have neither the length of experience nor a professional health or social care qualification are often appointed. Such qualifications are absolutely no guarantee of competence, but they do enhance confidence and provide a level of background knowledge that aid managers to discharge their responsibilities more effectively and assertively.

Chapter 2
Coping with Challenging Behaviour

I really don't like the phrase 'challenging behaviour' which started life as a non-pejorative term, 'behaviour that challenges services', and was intended to shift the focus away from people blaming service users for their dysfunctional conduct. Nowadays, it has degenerated into a rather clichéd expression that has negative connotations and has become almost synonymous with the derogatory language that was devised to replace such as 'disturbed' or 'agitated' behaviour. The principles of Positive Behavioural Support encourage us to think of antisocial or upsetting actions as being ways to express anger and distress, understanding such behaviours in humanistic and empathic ways rather than characterising them by the generalised, almost clinical term 'challenging behaviour'.

However, that phrase is prevalent in academic circles and throughout services; it is a shorthand term which everyone is familiar with so I shall reluctantly use it throughout this book.

One of the first research studies on the subject of the effect of challenging behaviour on carers was published in 1995, by Bromley and Emerson. The latter identified that carers experience a range of strong emotions when they are exposed to frequent and enduring behaviours, such as physical aggression, self-harm, prolonged shouting or screaming, destruction of property and personal items, inappropriate social behaviour, like stripping, faecal smearing or urinating in public places, running away and over activity.

Those emotions were notable for both their intensity and the frequency that they occurred. For instance, 'sadness' or 'annoyance' was reported as being felt by 38% and 41% of the group of carers that Bromley and Emerson questioned as a consequence to physical aggression. 'Sadness' was also experienced by 38% as a response to self-injury and 39% with regard to destructiveness. 'Despair' was experienced at a rate of 22%, 32% and 33% for, in turn, aggression, self-injury and destructiveness. Anger and fear were similarly strong emotions prevalent as a response to all three types of challenge, but more likely (24% and 19%) when carers were confronted with aggression. 'Disgust' was less common, but had a particular association with self-injury, with 15% of the study group reporting this as a feeling they had when they encountered this particular behaviour.

When I first read this article, two things struck me: the strength and intensity of the emotions that were experienced and the high proportion of respondents who acknowledged their occurrence. 'Disgust' and 'despair' are very powerful feelings which must be difficult to cope with. Also, as is revealed by the percentages, the different emotions were often experienced by more than a third of the study group.

My own experiences corroborate these findings in terms of the intensity and extremity of emotions that carers feel in these circumstances. Several times in my career I have had phone calls from normally resilient and assertive staff absolutely distraught, because, on that particular day, they are exhausted by someone's physical and aggressive behaviour and no longer have any idea of how to cope with it. I have seen carers become very incensed because service users have used foul, abusive and personal language towards them, or really angry because less able residents have been intimidated or attacked by their peers. Members of staff have confided in me about how frightened they were during certain traumatic incidents, describing the distressing physical phenomena, such as a racing heart rate or uncontrollable trembling that they felt. The emotions that carers endure are very real, intense and potentially damaging and hard to appreciate by colleagues who don't have the same experiences.

Bromley and Emerson also provided some insights regarding specific stressors related to challenging behaviour. They discovered that carers regard as stressful those behaviours which endure over a long period of time, that appear to be intractable and resistant to interventions or unpredictable and difficult to understand.

Unsurprisingly, staff members were more affected by challenging individuals with learning disabilities who harmed others or themselves; in particular, the physical size and strength of a service user were implicated as causes of apprehension and stress. The impact of aggressive service users on other clients was also a significant factor in affecting the wellbeing of members of staff.

There is a whole range of behaviours which are loosely described as 'socially inappropriate behaviour' which can affect carers in a negative way even though they do not entail physical peril. These include stripping, urinating in inappropriate places, including in public locations, running away, sudden, loud or repetitive vocalisations or persistently invading people's personal space.

Raczka (2005) gives some very specific examples of challenging behaviour revealed by the focus group of residential care home staff that he questioned. He described instances of staff having their hair pulled, being punched, slapped, and scratched or spat at. Self-injurious behaviour included eye gouging, hitting one's head against the floor or hand biting. Anti-social behaviour sometimes entailed inappropriate sexual contact, such as touching carers' breasts, as well as instances of being extremely noisy for long periods or 'temper tantrums'.

He also reports some extremely visceral reactions to the immediate experience of challenges, including feeling absolutely sick, the uncomfortable sensation of a racing heart rate, feeling very frightened or conscious of the need to control of the instinctive reaction to fight back and hit out at aggressive clients.

All the feelings that members of Raczka's focus group describe are perfectly in accordance with the effects of the secretion of adrenaline and the phenomenon of 'fight and flight'. Smith's Time Intensity Model helps us both to understand how these processes affect service users and explain the potential progress of an aggressive incident in terms of a 'trigger', a form of threat or frustration causing 'escalation' fuelled biochemically by adrenaline. Also, the model helps to explain the primitive feelings that members of staff encounter and the tensions that they endure in trying to master either anger or trepidation and act in a calm, facilitative manner. The secretion of adrenaline is associated with certain impairments of one's ability to communicate with others and process information, as well as the peripheral visual field, making the task of staff in dealing with challenges in an appropriate manner even more difficult.

Following the conclusion of an aggressive incident, it is probable that carers, just like service users will experience feelings of mental and physical exhaustion, and be low spirited or even tearful, whilst still continuing to provide support to their clients.

Research relating to the long-term effects of exposure to aggression or other forms of challenge cites feelings of guilt at letting down clients, embarrassment from a perception that colleagues regard one as being incompetent for not dealing with a situation effectively and losses in confidence. Other outcomes might include irritability, an unwarranted fear of the occurrence of further incidents or a decreased interest in work, even apathy.

In some areas, the use of removal and restraint techniques as a response to challenging behaviour is very frequent. Being restrained is very distressing for service users, but there is some research that carers who have to use these physical interventions are affected adversely. Performing the role of a lone worker supporting potentially volatile clients in their own flats is also a potent cause of anxiety.

Raczka (2005) gives some powerful examples of the real-life impact of challenges over time. People in the study refer to themselves lying awake at night, ruminating how they could have handled situations differently, having terrible headaches or flashbacks about being physically attacked. They also recount the onset of physical illness such as irritable bowel syndrome or depression and anxiety, requiring treatment by medication like Prozac. They talked as well about attempts at self-medication in the form of increased cigarette and alcohol intake.

Sometimes anguish generated by challenges can be more intellectual in nature. Whittington and Burns (2005) talk about the 'dilemmas' face by care staff who encounter challenges, the mental turmoil that staff experience trying to reconcile different perspectives like regarding behaviour as a form of communication or as a problem to be managed, or how to maintain boundaries, provide direction, whilst still being kind and respectful. Often carers feel that if they maintain boundaries and distance themselves from clients, this likely to be effective, but conflicts with the wish to appear sympathetic and supportive.

When carers are confronted by behaviour which is violent, disturbing or socially inappropriate, the precise feelings that they experience are dependent on the interpretation that they make as to the causes of behaviour and who is to blame. Carers might believe that they themselves are largely responsible for the behaviour, which they regard as preventable occurring and blame themselves for their apparent negligence. They might think that their lack of ability has contributed to challenges taking place, causing them to feel ashamed. Anger might be the outcome for carers who perceive service users to be wholly at fault for their problematic behaviour and believe that service users do things on purpose to annoy them. If carers believe that a particular behaviour is an inherent part of a learning-disabled person's nature, they might even experience a sense of despair (Cudre-Mauroux 2010). All these ways of attributing reasons for behaviour lead to strong, negative emotions which eat away at the self-esteem and emotional stability of carers and result in an increase in stress.

It is undoubtedly a common consequence of challenging behaviour is that carers make attributions, ascribe causes for aggressive or dysfunctional actions which are almost wholly negative. They assume that service users are totally in control of their behaviour, are doing things to personally annoy them and in order to be 'attention seeking' or 'manipulative'. These attitudes result in a lack of empathy and understanding towards clients and a failure to attain a greater awareness as to why people are behaving in such a way.

Primarily, service users are affected by this unsophisticated approach, because a true picture of the reasons for behaviour and the triggers that initiate aggressive response is no longer being sought. Opportunities are lost to make significant changes to the environment, to the demands that carers make and to arrange suitable treatments, making it inevitable that challenging behaviour continues. The decrease in positive interactions from carers contingent on negative attributions for behaviour contributes to the very perpetuation of that behaviour, a negative consequence principally for the service user, but also the people who support him or her.

These thought processes also indirectly affect staff morale and well-being. Because their responses have become ineffective and unempathetic, carers suffer the added stress of enduring challenges and feel powerless to change things in any way. If they blame service users for their behaviour, staff members are more likely to be angry and apathetic towards them. Instead of seeking practical and effective ways to help service users, which focus on understanding the functionality of behaviours in an objective but sympathetic manner, staff are trapped in a cycle of negativity, recrimination and anger which is almost as damaging to them as to service users.

Carers who are regularly faced with aggressive or dysfunctional behaviour can be offered helpful support and guidance at several junctures. They can be given training which helps them to understand the significance of individual triggers for aggression and the importance of documenting and knowing early warning signs that a service user is becoming angry. Both triggers and early warning signs can be very idiosyncratic and sometimes obscure. For instance, people may be affected by noise, tiredness, intrusion of others or hunger all of which are readily understood and inferred by supporting staff. However, other precipitants for aggression might be much more subtle, such as specific words which may not have any connotations that give a clue that they are distressing, the presence of bright lighting or the impact of the symptoms associated with a serious mental disorder like schizophrenia, such as voices saying hurtful or upsetting things.

People who have learning disabilities, like anyone else, become angry for reasons which are specific to the individual and potential causes have to be learnt, documented and disseminated throughout the entire team, including new, inexperienced and temporary staff who have had less time to become acquainted with service users and significant items of information such as these.

Indicators that someone is losing his temper might be very overt like pacing, a louder voice, a raised fist or obviously angry expression. Often, they are much more subtle. Someone I knew, possibly because he had autism, developed a rather inane fixed smile when he first he started feeling upset. Another person would just tap her foot very slightly whilst someone else may start repeating a seemingly innocuous word incessantly. As with triggers for aggression, early indicators of losing one's temper are often very specific to the individual. Frequently it is possible to learn which early warning signs are likely to be displayed first, giving supporters more time to start investigating what has cause the service user to become distressed and try to address those factors.

When faced by someone who appears to be becoming aggressive, it is inevitable that carers will feel tense, fearful or annoyed due to the effects of adrenaline secretion, an automatic response that the body makes when we encounter a situation which is potentially threatening. This process diminishes people's ability to understand others, including the distressed service user, to express themselves effectively and to think clearly. Carers may be affected by the impact of adrenaline in ways that they find difficult to observe in themselves during an aggressive incident: their body posture may become unwittingly confrontational. Similarly, their facial expression or voice tone, volume and pitch may send messages of aggression, because they haven't been able to adequately control these aspects of non-verbal communication. These deficiencies in communication may add to the conflict in aggressive situations making them less easy to resolve with adverse, stressful consequences for both service users and carers.

Team members are helped by training that gives them the opportunity to learn about these phenomena, to become more aware about their demeanour and general communication when confronted by aggression and encourages them to develop a personal strategy for coping with potentially violent incidents. This exercise might entail individuals confronting aspects of service users' behaviour which specifically upset them and acknowledging their vulnerabilities. For instance, one person might be especially affected by spitting, whilst a colleague might be inordinately angered by verbal abuse. Another person might be distressed by faecal smearing whilst someone else might be angered by aggression towards other service users.

Carers might need not only to learn what constitutes appropriate body language, voice tone, pitch and level and facial expression as class-based teaching exercises, but also to practise these skills in simulated situations.

Other areas where education may be beneficial might include very specific training relating to specific conditions which affect service users, such as personality disorders, schizophrenia, autism, epilepsy, Fragile X and the impact of abuse. By gaining knowledge of these conditions where relevant to individual clients, carers are less likely to make negative attributions that are unhelpful to the service user, impair staff client relationships and diminish the ability to offer proactive support which is both beneficial to service users and which, by offering active solutions based on objective knowledge, is more likely to reduce carers' stress levels.

The support that people receive immediately after aggressive incidents is very important. Whenever carers are asked what they would like in these circumstances, they usually say that they want a few minutes away from the work situation, an opportunity to calm down, to collect their thoughts or even vent their feelings in privacy. People use those few minutes of relief in various diverse ways: one person might use it to get a bit of fresh air in the garden, another might have a cigarette, someone else might seek some time for himself in a quiet room or conversely wish for the support of a colleague to talk things through. Having the opportunity to use five minutes in any way that is suitable for that individual to recover from an incident does not seem an outrageous demand to me.

Also, carers appreciate genuine expressions of concern, particularly if they are articulated by members of the management team, which demonstrate warmth and sincerity. Someone who has been the primary focus of an aggressive incident prefers not to be harangued by requests to complete accident forms straightaway or to reflect in detail concerning the rights and wrongs of how the incident was handled immediately after its conclusion. Treatment for physical injuries should be expedited immediately entailing the provision of transport to the local accident and emergency centre if necessary. People who are really distressed should be given the opportunity to go home, again with transport arranged as far as possible.

When someone has had a very upsetting encounter causing sufficient emotional or physical trauma to warrant him or her taking sick leave, however brief, all effort must be made to maintain contact with that person and he or she will need sensitive support on return to work. A phased return may be appropriate. Certainly, each person who returns to work after a difficult incident should be offered the opportunity for further support and discussions related to the aggressive incident.

This type of post incident support is not the sole responsibility of the management team; it is most effective when all members of the work force understand the need for and readily participate in supporting their colleagues both immediately after an incident and subsequently.

Of course, support for staff should not simply consist of a reactive immediate response to individual incidents. Carers may experience feelings similar to those who have been characterised as suffering Post Traumatic Stress Disorder, if they have been subjected to severe violence or even if they endure constant exposure to minor forms of aggression or other challenges.

Reported phenomena include irritability, an unwarranted expectation that aggression will occur, flashbacks and a startled response to sudden noises or other disquieting events. They may seek to cope with the memory of difficult episodes with service users by actively seeking interactions that make it more likely that they will experience similar encounters. Alternatively, they may avoid those situations or service users whom they regard as threatening. Emotions such as anger, fear, self-recrimination and resentment, against colleagues and managers as well as clients, may endure over a significant period of time. People may lose their sense of self-esteem, because they blame themselves for an incident occurring or reprimand themselves for failures to anticipate and deal effectively with aggression. They may become depressed, apathetic, lose interest in their work and contribute less.

It is not inevitable that staff will feel all these insidious and damaging emotions. The general culture of the entire team and approach of managers are highly significant factors in preventing their occurrence. A simple recognition of how distressing it is to be regularly exposed to challenges, even if they are not obviously harmful as in the case of repetitive speech and constant loud vocalisations and a demonstration of empathic understanding are good foundations, particularly when someone has just returned to work after an especially upsetting incident.

However, team members and bosses can be supportive in practical ways by ensuring that their traumatised colleagues do not immediately resume working with clients who have harmed them but are gradually reintroduced. Co-workers can encourage them to have regular breaks and observe for any signs of stress, intervening in a sympathetic and helpful way.

Practical support could entail providing specific training for individuals which address deficits in their learning and development. For instance, people who have been the focus of challenges may need help to develop a self-management plan to deal with specific scenarios. They may need to learn about the triggers and early warning signs appertaining to individual clients or guidance on what constitutes effective proactive support that minimises challenges developing in the first place. They may benefit from detailed knowledge about service users' histories and the clinical conditions which contribute to challenges, such as autism, specific psychiatric disorders or Fragile X.

Managers have a specific role to play in providing formal structures of support like monthly one to one supervision sessions, which give an opportunity for staff to discuss their progress with respect to challenges and facilitating Personal Development Plans which capture the sort of learning needs previously alluded to and maps a way forward to address those deficits.

Formal structures are very important as a means of guaranteeing that support is given in an individualised and structured manner. Nevertheless, leaders and colleagues must never underestimate the value of offering informal support on a daily basis if necessary, by providing encouragement, giving opportunities to reflect on prevailing difficulties and progress and anticipating any stressful incidents.

It may be that the distress that team members have undergone cannot simply be dealt with through these types of internal processes and they require specialised counselling provided by an external practitioner, a service that organisations that deliver care services should make available for their employees when it is necessary.

There may be compelling reasons why aggressive incidents or indeed any traumatic work event might have a proportionally greater impact than be expected. Breakwell

(1997) describes five factors which might influence how a carer deals subsequently with the after-effects of problematic behaviour:

> ➢ The presence of concomitant life stressors – such as financial problems, relationship difficulties, bereavements or illness experienced by self or a family member.
> ➢ Having a depressive mindset – people who have such a cognitive approach are more likely to believe that being subjected to assaults is an integral part of a succession of events that they have no control over
> ➢ Lack of social support networks – people who have limited support from friends and family have less opportunities to talk about incidents and so are less likely to resolve the tensions arising from such events
> ➢ Believing that victims of aggression fit certain stereotypes – i.e. they are people who attract that sort of behaviour because they are authoritarian, provocative or incompetent. It is very easy for someone who has experienced aggressive events to appropriate that stereotype and revile themselves for their perceived inadequacies.
> ➢ Self-esteem is mainly achieved via work – if people with this mind-set experience traumatic incidents, they are bound to affect them more than carers who have a more rounded lifestyle

Cudre-Mauroux (2010) talks about the concept of 'self-efficacy', the perception of one's ability to deal with certain demands and its significance for professional care givers in helping them to manage their stress levels in response to challenging behaviour. Low self-efficacy is characterised by negative thoughts towards both service users and the general context, inability to control one's emotions, perception of failure to due to personal weaknesses and the attributes of service users and a failure to persevere in finding solutions to difficulties.

The perception of high self-efficacy is associated with a positive outlook to challenges, an ability to regulate and master negative thoughts and emotions, the belief that it is possible to access necessary resources and the presence of attributions for behaviour which are external i.e. that concede that the causes for challenging behaviour are largely beyond the control of the service user. Carers who have this mind-set feel empowered and confident that they will be effective, so inherently reduce their stress levels whilst also having a more helpful, empathetic regard for service users.

Generally, for both the welfare of service users and the stress levels of carers, it is beneficial that the latter feel capable, have recourse to strategies and solutions and a sense of optimism that those approaches will eventually prevail. How can such a mind-set be nurtured? After all the common wisdom is that challenges endure over many years and even if they do become less frequent there is always a possibility that they will re-emerge if those people who historically displayed aggressive or socially unacceptable behaviour are exposed to new stressors. Carers who support individuals with learning disabilities who are dysfunctional need qualities of tenacity, resilience, assertiveness and positivity about both their abilities and their clients. However, to effectively help others they also need skills and knowledge which can bolster the use of practical, objective and evidence based coping styles rather than those that are emotional and reactive.

Some measures have been developed to assess staff attitudes towards service users who challenge. These include the Attributional Style Questionnaire (Dagnan and Hill 2012) which asks participants to look at two scenarios which present the same challenge with unnamed and then named participants and identify possible reasons for behaviour.

The Shortened Ways of Coping – Revised Questionnaire (SWC-R), devised by Hatton and Emerson (1994) seeks to measure the use of two coping styles: 'wishful thinking' which entails coping with the feelings engendered by a stressful event whilst not attempting to alter the situation, often leading to negative outcomes and distress for service users; 'practical coping', addressing challenges by attempting to find solutions and seeking changes in the environment and levels of demands, an approach associated with more positive results for both services users and carers, including an increased level of job satisfaction for the latter.

Conversely, the Promotion of Acceptance in Carers and Teachers tool devised by Noone and Hastings (2010) encourages participants to accept the causes of stress without feeling that there should always be ready solution.

An essential process for ensuring that we fully understand why people have behaved in a certain manner and to improve how they are supported is some form of critical analysis after serious incidents, during which carers seek to answer key questions such as what happened during the incident, why people think it happened, what were the triggers and how approaches could be improved in the future. Aside from its main purpose of attempting to develop more effective ways to support service users, this type of exercise can be very therapeutic for carers in terms of either developing appreciation of triggers and effective ways to mitigate their impact, thus making it less likely that challenging behaviour will occur, or assuring them in some circumstances their support could not be faulted or generally reassuring them that a problem solving approach is being used.

As well as ensuring that service users are okay when they have been subjected to any physical intervention, whether breakaway techniques or removal and restraint techniques, support should be given routinely to members of staff who have had to employ such measures, not simply because of the physical dimension, but also because of the potentiality for staff feeling a whole range of emotions such as guilt, anxiety, fear which may remain with them if not addressed and discussed. Also, it is important to monitor that physical interventions have been used correctly to ensure that the likelihood of staff using practices which might lead to any form of criticism and sanction is minimised.

Staff who assist people who possibly may challenge in community setting like supported living project where they work by themselves, especially need to be supported with care, with a system being in place whereby carers can readily access support by telephone or be relieved in exceptional circumstances. In these scenarios where staff could readily feel very isolated, post incident support and debriefing becomes even more urgent and must be promptly and actively provided.

Ian's story, an example of how carers can be helped to have a more positive view about someone that they regard as challenging:

Ian had lived in long stay hospitals since he was a ten-year-old boy. He moved to a new care home for people with learning disabilities and mental health needs when he was in his late thirties. He displayed a plethora of challenging behaviours including destroying his own property, urinating on his bedding, cutting himself, shouting and swearing, hitting members of staff and pulling their hair. He would usually exhibit at least one of these behaviours every single day, causing his carers to become very tense, and sometimes angry with Ian.

All the team attended a meeting facilitated by members of the local Community Learning Disabilities Team during which they explored the reasons why Ian behaved as he did. It clearly emerged from examining history and constructing a timeline that he had been severely sexually abused by other residents when he was a young lad, which had cause him lasting emotional distress. Although it was not possible to discover all the reasons for his challenges and make swift progress in addressing his problem behaviours, identifying that traumatic aspect of his past was sufficient to help carers feel more empathic towards Ian rather than perpetually annoyed by him, with a resultant improvement in mutual relationships and a much less stressful working environment.

Sebastian and Julie illustrates the importance of critical review to ascertain why incidents occur (avoiding unwarranted self-recrimination

Sebastian had lived in his current care home, a specialised service for people with complex needs and learning disabilities, for three years. Although when he first lived there, he had very angry outbursts virtually each day, gradually through the application of Positive Behavioural Support principles he had developed astonishingly well to the extent that plans were being made with him for him to live in his own flat in a different part of the city. He had an appointment to have an eye test one Saturday morning, a busy time of the day, but no different to many other situations that he had encountered successfully in the previous few years. Unfortunately, Sebastian became very angry at the opticians, tipping over displays in the shop and kicking waste bins in the shopping precinct, causing no damage but alarming both the general public and Julie, the carer who was accompanying him. Julie and her colleague, who had been summoned to help, gave Sebastian excellent support and he was able to calm down quite rapidly and return home.

Julie was extremely distressed and blamed herself for the incident, as there was no obvious trigger for its occurrence. She was given sensitive support which included her having some time away from service users to help her settle. We did a very brief analysis of the incident, and I was able to reassure her that, on the face of it, it did not appear that she contributed to Sebastian becoming angry. We did a much more detailed and comprehensive debriefing a couple of days later by which time we ascertained that Sebastian had been muttering 'laugh at me, laugh at me' whilst ascending the optician's stairs. This recollection and information provided by his mother that he had been cruelly teased the last time that he wore glasses when he was a boy, helped to reassure Julie that she had not been neglectful or unobservant and should not blame herself for the incident occurring. This account demonstrates the value of post incident analysis as a means to allay negative and ill-founded emotions experienced by carers as well as the primary aim of establishing the reasons for behaviours happening.

Paula and Carol (the significance of humour as a coping strategy)

Ashley went out with Paula and Carol to a local park. Because he has severe epilepsy and autism, sometimes Ashley would act in an unusual and impulsive manner as was the case this time when he suddenly stripped off his clothes during his walk, probably due to a complex partial seizure. He instantly ran away from Paula and Carol, fortunately in the direction of a small wood. Although there was nobody in the immediate vicinity, obviously the two ladies were extremely perturbed by this scenario and its potential for compromising Ashley's dignity, exposing him to voyeurism and causing them embarrassment. They ran after him and eventually caught up with him, using one of their coats to cover him up, even though supporting Ashley so closely put them at risk of being hit or pinched by him. They succeeded in helping him to get dressed before returning home.

When they returned both of them were rather shaken by this experience, but were quickly able to see its funny side, recounting the story in the office. There are perils in this response to challenging incidents: carers could be seen to be disrespectful towards service users and laughing at them. Degenerating into 'gallows humour' can be a sign of cynicism and a blunting of emotional responses. However, Paula and Carol's reaction absolutely did not accord with either of these unhelpful approaches; their amusement was derived principally from their self-derogatory perception of how ridiculous they probably looked to an uninformed onlooker, laboriously chasing after a naked young man. Adopting a humorous view of what could have been a distressing and dangerous situation, but one that they were able to avert, was a good way to relieve the stress associated with the event.

Alan's story (Illustrating how learning from experience in a way which informs future practice can be a helpful coping strategy)

One evening I was congratulating myself for the progress that Paul had made as he had had no instances of inappropriate physical contact with other service users for several months. The very next morning I received a phone call that Paul had seriously attacked James who sustained severe scratches and disfiguring abrasions to his face. This had happened late in the evening when an alarm should have been set to alert the one waking night staff who was on duty that Paul had exited his flat, a practice that I had ceased to affirm should be followed at all times.

Both service users' families were distressed by this incident and its consequences; Paul's family were distressed by the stigmatisation caused by his actions and ultimately felt that he should no longer live in his current accommodation, whilst James' parents were upset by the highly visible injuries sustained by their son. Both parties felt, understandably, that the situation could have been avoided.

Personally, I felt very guilty for assuming that the progress someone had made would mean that he would never harm anyone again we could afford to relax our approaches. I blamed myself for the incident, James' injuries, the increase in Paul's negative reputation and the anguish felt by both families.

Obviously, continuing to feel so distraught was ultimately not very helpful for me as an individual and as the manager of a care home for people with learning disabilities and complex needs, whose residents and staff still needed support and leadership. The things that helped me cope with my feelings were initially the loyalty and understanding of my colleagues. Ultimately though, learning from the experience, appreciating that even small omissions of support and lapses in concentration can have cataclysmic consequences for service users, that one should never become complacent, were the most effective ways of reconciling the emotions engendered by this incident.

Kyle and Lee's story
When Kyle came to live at his new home, having previously lived at his parents' home, it took a while for people to understand him. Often, he would have very

explosive outbursts during which he would charge at members of staff attempting to hit, kick or bite them. Gradually his team learnt that the outbursts could be anticipated by an understanding of Kyle's triggers and the early warning signs of his behaviour. Also, people developed a 'low arousal' approach which was helpful since Kyle had a condition called Fragile X which meant that he became excitable and irritable quite quickly.

Although the frequency and intensity of Kyle's incidents definitely reduced, Lee, one of his care staff remained very anxious about him, particularly when he was working in the evenings when there were less staff around.

Lee found it helpful to talk about his fears openly without fear of criticism. We analysed reports of Lyle's incidents and were able to agree that these hardly ever happened during the evening, partly because the team adopted a low arousal approach in which they ensured that levels of lighting and noise levels were reduced, and they monitored their own interactions with Kyle to ensure that these were not over stimulating. Also, he was actively encouraged to wind down during the evening by having a long, hot, and relaxing bath and listen to music in his room rather than engaging too much with others.

This process of reflection helped Lee to become less stressed in several ways. He was able to appreciate that Kyle's behaviour tended to occur in certain contexts and was less likely in the evening when it was quieter and less stimulating and so his anxiety concerning the likelihood of incidents happening at the time was unwarranted. He also was more readily able to understand that he and the team had developed extremely effective approaches which helped to ensure that Kyle remained calm and content. Furthermore, he learnt more about the impact of Kyle's condition, Fragile X, and was able to readily relate the latter's potential challenges to a condition that Kyle had no control over, increasing Lee's understanding, empathy levels and positive approach towards Kyle.

Chapter 3
Coping with Service Users' Characteristics

We live in an age when physical attractiveness is celebrated constantly by such media as advertising, reality television programmes, cinema and the general culture of celebrity.

History and literature are punctuated by expressions of opinions in which the humanity of people with learning disabilities is denied. Often a link is established between the person's subhuman nature and their physical appearance, habits and characteristics. Here is an account written by Martin Luther, the Christian theologian of the fifteenth century who fathered Protestantism, which describes an encounter with a child who has a learning disability in which he finds the child's characteristics to be highly objectionable, literally demonises him and recommends death as a solution:

'Eight years ago, there was one in Dessau whom I, Martinus Luther, saw and grappled with. He was twelve years old, had the use of his eyes and all his senses, so that one might think he was a normal child. But he did nothing but gorge himself as much as four peasants or threshers. He ate, defecated, and drooled and, if anyone tackled him, he screamed. If things didn't go well, he wept. So I said to the Prince of Anhalt: "If I were the Prince, I should take the child to the Moldau River which flows near Dessau and drown him." But the Prince of Anhalt and the Prince of Saxony, who happened to be present, refused to follow my advice. Thereupon, I said, "Well, then the Christians shall order the Lord's Prayer to be said in church and pray that the dear

Lord take the Devil away." This was done daily in Dessau and the changeling died in the following year'.

The following words were written over a hundred years ago by someone who contributed to framing of the Mental Deficiency Act of 1913, legislation that led to the segregation of many people with learning disabilities from the rest of the community in Britain and is full of beliefs and opinions that few of us would agree with nowadays.

'They come into the world without even the hereditary instinct of sucking. As they grow up they have to be fed, and would die of inanition amid abundance of food were it not put into their mouths. If they are conscious of excessive heat or cold, they are devoid of any idea of the remedy. They respire, assimilate, and excrete, but they have no sexual instinct, and cannot reproduce their degenerate species. They may be capable of inarticulate cries, but they cannot speak. They possess the power of muscular movement, but locomotion is absent. They have eyes, but they see not; ears, but they hear not; they have no intelligence and no consciousness of pleasure or pain; in fact, their mental state is one entire negation. The short existence of most of these creatures is spent in bed, where they lie huddled up in an ante-natal posture. They are hideous, repulsive creatures whom Nature permits to enter, but not to linger, in the world'
(Tredgold 1908)

A year later, Sir James Crichton-Brown, giving evidence before the 1908 Royal Commission on the Care and Control of the Feeble-Minded, recommended the compulsory sterilisation of those with learning disabilities and mental illness, describing them as "our social rubbish" which should be "swept up and garnered and utilised as far as possible". He went on to complain, "We pay much attention to the breeding of our horses, our cattle, our dogs and poultry, even our flowers and vegetables; surely it's not too much to ask that a little care be bestowed upon the breeding and rearing of our race". Crichton-Brown was in distinguished company. In a memo to the prime minister in 1910, Winston Churchill cautioned "the multiplication of the feeble-minded is a very terrible danger to the race".

Supporters of eugenics in Parliament included the Labour MP Will Crooks who described disabled people as "like human vermin" who "crawl about doing absolutely nothing, except polluting and corrupting everything they touch".

Modern views regarding people with learning disabilities may not be expressed in such an extreme and derogatory way, but a recent study reveals a great deal of negativity towards this client group.

67% of the British public feel uncomfortable talking to disabled people.

36% of people tend to think of disabled people as not as productive as everyone else.

85% of the British public believe that disabled people face prejudice.

24% of disabled people have experienced attitudes or behaviours where other people expected less of them because of their disability.

21% of 18–34-year-olds admit that they have actually avoided talking to a disabled person because they weren't sure how to communicate with them.

Disabled people and their families tell Scope that negative attitudes affect every area of their lives – in the playground, at work, in shops, on the street.

But how can we improve attitudes to disabled people?

Much of the discomfort people feel about disability may stem from a lack of understanding.

We live in an age when we feel superior to these historical figures and think we are immune from developing such views. Nevertheless, there are many recent instances which illustrate circumstances in which carers somehow lose sight of what constitutes basic moral decency and treat people with learning disabilities as if they were less than human. However, thoughts about the utter dependency of people with very profound disabilities and the apparent meaninglessness of their lives must occasionally pass through the minds of even the most dedicated carers.

This process may occur because of characteristics displayed by some service users which mark them out as being different, annoying or distasteful in some way.

It is not my intention to be disrespectful to any person who has a learning disability. However, those who have severe and profound disabilities, autism and significant communication deficits are not always the easiest or most comfortable to support at times. They may be doubly incontinent, need to wear protective pads, and have to be changed regularly, not an easy or pleasant task especially if the service user is an adult.

As well as encountering faeces and urine on a daily basis, carers may have to deal with menstrual blood, mucous, sputum, dribbling saliva, vomit or semen. Handling bodily waste or fluids is unpleasant, particularly if it is an inevitable daily aspect of one's job role, which relentlessly reoccurs and has to be confronted by carers each shift.

Sometimes, there might be factors that make a member of staff less able to cope with the sights and smells associated with caring for someone who has no control of their bodily waste. They may be sick or weary due to a prolonged spell of work; someone who normally is relatively easy to wash, and change might suddenly become more difficult one day because he or she is feeling unwell. A member of staff who usually can cope with normal faecal and urinary waste might find it difficult to handle diarrhoea or the odour associated with urinary tract infections.

People who have profound learning disabilities may sometimes have increased muscle tone and are hard to manoeuvre when carers are delivering essential personal care. Sometimes the disabled person's body shape and rigidity limit the effectiveness of moving and handling aids, throwing greater reliance on manual handling by staff. Others may have a degree of involuntary limb movement, again making dressing, washing and other aspects of personal care arduous.

Service users may have habits and behaviours which, although not challenging as such, are hard to deal with over a long period of time. For instance, they may have characteristic, highly repetitive vocalisations, regurgitate, smear or flick mucous and sputum.

People with profound disabilities invariably have extremely limited abilities to communicate in any but the simplest of forms. This lack of reciprocity, the inability to give much back to carers in the form of communication can be very dispiriting over a period of time, as can be the seemingly impossible prospect of those service users developing in any way.

During the past twenty-five years, the concept of Person-Centred Planning has evolved within the learning-disabled community and those who provide services and care for that group of people. At the heart of this concept is the notion that any support an individual receives should be informed entirely by that person's wishes and needs and no one should have to fit in with the routines and requirements a service.

Several Person Centred tools have been devised which serve to an approach which appears on obvious way to support people but is still relatively novel: Essential Lifestyle Plans (ELP) capture among many other things, the aspects of life that are essential for an individual, their likes and dislikes and dreams; a PATH (Planning Alternative Tomorrows with Hope) aspires to graphically delineate the dreams and aspirations of individuals as part of a dynamic process involving informal and family networks of support which seeks to help people with learning disabilities achieve those dreams and aspirations; a MAP (Making Action Plans) is another highly visual format which acknowledges difficult aspects a person's life ('nightmares') but focuses on principally the positives such as dreams and gifts.

All these approaches share common themes like concentrating on what people can do rather than their deficits, their gifts and abilities, placing the person and his/her needs at the heart of care and support planning and affirming that people with learning disabilities have the capacity to develop as much as anyone else.

Champions of Person-Centred Planning strongly affirm the principle that it is an approach that should be applied to everyone regardless of their level of disability. In fact, the aforementioned ELP format was devised as a means to gather knowledge and inform planning for those individuals who were leaving long stay institutions in the 1990s who did not have the ability to communicate their needs and wishes and about whom there was an extreme paucity of information due to inadequate documentation during their time in hospital.

The principal beneficiaries of this radical and novel change of approach are of course those people for whom it was devised. However, the PCP methodology enhances carers' perspectives of the people that they support by prompting them to see beyond how individuals present externally, to look for their gifts and capacities and regard them as developing individuals irrespective of the severity of someone's cognitive impairment.

Janet's story

Janet went to live in a long stay hospital when she was about four or five. She was born with a severe learning disability and some type of ophthalmological infection that necessitated the removal of her eye tissue when she was just a few days old. She never physically developed, remaining the size of a seven-year-old child throughout her adult life, presenting a disconcerting sight because she was quite emaciated and of course had empty sunken sockets where her eye would have been. Until the age of fifty-two she would not tolerate wearing clothes for any period longer than a few minutes, sometimes stripping herself within seconds of being dressed. She had no speech over than indistinct vocalisations and often was irritable when approached by staff, lashing out or scratching them. As she would not wear clothing, she could not remain in communal areas and was largely confined to her own barren room. Also, she was frequently doubly incontinent and developed medical conditions which caused her to vomit often. People who cared for Janet considered her a difficult person with whom to spend any length of time, sometimes finding her repugnant due to her incontinence, vomiting, nudity, aggression and unusual physical appearance.

A programme was put in place to desensitise Janet from adverse feelings of wearing clothes and she gradually started accepting being dressed for reasonable periods of time. Her team instigated a toilet training regime which was successful and were able to secure effective treatment for her illnesses, so that she hardly vomited at all. She was able to start sitting with other people, tolerate items in her room and even go for drives. Gradually her tolerance to new experiences increased and the likelihood that she would take her clothes off diminished so that she was able to go on holiday to conventional settings and eventually moved to a small care home in the suburbs of Bristol.

As Janet's quality of life improved so in tandem did the positive view of staff increase and she was no longer someone that they found stressful and unpleasant to support.

Janet's story illustrates the importance of discovering a person's individuality and personality whilst ensuring his or her basic human rights to dignity and opportunities to develop. Without these processes it was difficult for staff to relate to her as a human being with a consequent effect on their own stress level and feelings of well-being.

Another aspect of people with learning disabilities which can cause stress for members of staff is the levels of stimulation within the environment with which individuals can cope and the tensions caused by differences particularly for people living in a communal setting.

Often disabled people who also have autism find a highly stimulating environment which is noisy and busy to be very uncomfortable to the point of being unbearable. The injurious impact of sensory phenomena such as noise, light and general 'busyness' of a living or working area is frequently difficult to appreciate, especially if someone doesn't have the ability to express their discomfort in words.

It is useful for carers to seek the views of people that can explain how they feel when assailed with apparently normal sensory stimuli. Here are some quotes from people with autism who can verbally articulate their experiences:

Light touch feels like a cattle prod
(Grandin)

I was also frightened of the vacuum cleaner, the food mixer and the liquidiser because they sounded about five times as loud as they actually were.
(White)

Sometimes when other kids spoke to me, I would scarcely hear, then sometimes they sounded like bullets.
(White)

Hearing gets louder sometimes… Things seem suddenly closer sometimes. Sometimes things get suddenly brighter
(Oliver)

It is reasonable to assume that many people with severe learning disabilities who cannot express themselves with any degree of clarity have similar perceptions of the world and carers have to constantly bear this in mind and moderate their tone of voice, ensure that background noise is minimal, be mindful that they are not too near, avoid excessive touch, consider the need to dim lighting and make certain that their body movements are not too intrusive. However, those residents who prefer a low arousal, muted environment might be sharing a home with people who are exuberant and outgoing, who prefer a much more stimulating mode of interaction. Strain is imposed on those who support people with such a disparate view of the sensory world and interactions because carers constantly need to adjust their approaches on a day to day basis and also have to reconcile the tensions caused by people with different outlooks and perceptions living together in close proximity.

Andrew was in the process of being supported to move into a flat having lived in a care home for seven years. Although this was a desire that he had expressed for many years, despite the efforts of the team that supported him, it proved very difficult to make swift progress with this aim, mainly because of difficulties in securing a social worker and also a subsequent reluctance on the part of social services to commit to supporting his move to his own place.

Andrew was determined to move to his own flat, so much so that when the lease was secured, he insisted on moving in straight away, leaving the care home that he lived at for five years before his team could properly assess the hazards associated with his new living environment and transition.

He had severe epilepsy which made it likely that he would have a seizure of some sort every day and so had funding for one to one support, which continued when he left residential care.

However, the small flat that he now lived in was quite different to his accommodation where his supporting staff were able to go to other areas of the building so that Andrew didn't feel that he was being monitored all the time and had some personal space. The only options that his personal assistants could pursue to avoid the latter were to go into the sleeping room or leave the flat for a short while. Sometimes Andrew was unsure whether he wanted that personal space or whether he wanted his carers to remain in his vicinity to ensure that he was safe.

Other stressors included his step-father being ill, confusion in his mind about the appropriate dose that he could take of one of his epilepsy 'rescue' medications and developing a chest infection. Of course, the transition itself, which had been deferred so often in the past, adjusting to his new routine and his habitual poor mental health were also contributing factors.

After several weeks, Andrew was involved in a serious incident in which he struck and racially abused a member of staff. The police were called, and he was arrested and charged. During one of his police interviews, he struck a female member of staff. When he returned home, he refused support from his team and was very low spirited, saying things like 'I don't care whether I live or die'.

With sensitive support, after a few days he accepted support again, treatment for his chest infection was initiated and his moodily gradually improved.

However, the team that supported him were left quite traumatised by the events. Many people, especially the person who had been racially abused, felt very angry towards Andrew, or were anxious about resuming supporting him. People also developed feelings of extreme anxiety that he might harm himself or suffer a severe epileptic seizure in the period that he was refusing support. There were worries that ultimately, he might need to be detained involuntarily in a Psychiatric Treatment and Assessment Centre if his mental health became worse. Also, his carers felt that they had failed very badly in allowing the situation to deteriorate that he had become so challenging and police involvement was necessitated.

Perhaps the most traumatising aspect of this episode was the impact of Andrew's extremely unpleasant racial abuse on both the person it was aimed at and his colleagues. Notwithstanding a physical attack on the same person and a female colleague later that day whilst he was at the police station, it was the racial slurs about which everyone was most upset. Coming from someone who hadn't ever showed any racist tendencies whatsoever and who had a good relationship with his victim his misdemeanour seemed both inexplicable and inexcusable given his extremely mild learning disability and the perception that he must surely have understood how offensive his comments were.

It is not likely that immediate support given in these circumstances would quickly result in someone who has been racially abused overcoming the feelings that they might have and becoming reconciled to the service user who has victimised him. Certain things definitely are helpful though. The member of staff certainly should not be expected to continue working with someone that has been so abusive to him. Also, opportunity must be given at the earliest opportunity for the person who has been abused to express his feelings concerning the incident to whomever he feels most comfortable. Such emotions are not likely to be dissipated rapidly and further debriefing may be needed. Certainly, someone who has been abused in this way would want to be assured that the incident was taken seriously by his colleagues and at all levels of the organisation. It would be that person's right to press charges and he may want to pursue that course of action, not necessarily in the spirit of retribution, but rather to feel that the matter has been dealt with in a fair and just way.

The person should not be expected to readily forgive the person that has abused them. However, as a way of sublimating feelings of anger and resentment, in the scenario delineated above it may be helpful for a colleague that the abused person trusts to facilitate reflection on the factors which might have caused Andrew to become so angry that he became so offensive. However, this should not be forced on the member of staff and he should only be encouraged to follow process when he is absolutely ready.

A potent source of distress for carers who are black or belong to an ethnic minority is being subjected to racist language and attitudes. Usually, staff who have this experience are extremely forbearing and understanding, being very willing to excuse such behaviour as part of lack of understanding on the part of the perpetrator, the influence of parents and limited opportunities to learn appropriate and respectful attitudes towards people from other cultures.

At the very least colleagues should recognise that racist comments are potentially hurtful and damaging even though generally the objects of such abuse generally 'laugh it off', and ensure that each episode is acknowledged, staff are given comfort and support and the opportunity to have some time away from supporting the individual in question.

Such incidents should never be ignored or regarded as being impossible to address because of the limited abilities someone with a learning disability might have. It is indeed the case, as victims of verbal abuse often aver, that service users racist attitudes are a result of poor role modelling and lack of education and so on every occasion that an incident of this type occurs there should be some form of debriefing with the relevant service user which seeks to help the latter understand that his or her behaviour or words are deeply offensive. However, especially if the person finds it difficult to learn, a structured programme of education should be pursued irrespective of whether a racist event has taken place, using easy read or pictorial formats if appropriate.

We must never assume that someone who is repeatedly subjected to racist abuse and generally appears to cope with it quite well is not hurt by offensive comments. Regular exposure to these episodes could be extremely damaging and those experiencing them for a prolonged time should receive ongoing support at a formal level from managers, who should also ensure that all racist incidents are documented so that colleagues at all levels are aware of the extent of the problem. When new appointments are made staff should be made aware that they may be subjected to a degree of racial abuse, with the reassurance that they will be given appropriate support and education will continue to be provided to abusive service users

Some form of professional counselling may be helpful in these circumstances, but many staff are sustained very effectively by the concern shown by their immediate colleagues and the ongoing support, both moral and practical that they offer.

A similar structured approach to service user education and victim support may need to be employed when carers are subjected to offensive comments about body image, appearance and weight or approaches which are rooted in chauvinism and sexism. As with racism, people subjected to abuse readily dismiss these phenomena as aspects of lack of cognitive ability and dysfunctional upbringing, but similarly they always should be taken seriously by colleagues and no assumptions made that the person subjected to abuse has not be hurt.

It is absolutely necessary that all accusations made by service users are investigated to the highest degree of stringency. The history of support of people with learning disabilities has been bedevilled until very recently by negligent approaches which often resulted in failure to acknowledge and fully investigate accusations made by recipients of care.

Nevertheless, there are sometimes individuals who have a history of making false accusations. If this appertains, with a consistent history of staff being completely exonerated, the situations when such false accusations may be made should be fully documented. A strategy should be evolved with senior managers and external authorities which minimises the likelihood that the full investigatory process will be followed on every single occasion that an accusation is made if it is really likely, given the service user's history, that the accusation will prove to be unfounded.

Chapter 4
Coping with Death and Loss

Donald went to live in Stoke Park Hospital, as a young boy, before he was even ten. His mother had died and his father, who regularly changed his location due to his position in the army, felt that he could no longer look after him.

As Donald grew up, he developed a reputation for being mischievous and adventurous which was nurtured by the many anecdotes that could be heard about him. He regularly found ways to travel on the train to London and other places in England without paying, usually being intercepted by the Transport Police at his destination, who would then contact his care team so that he could be retrieved from whatever distant place he had ended up.

There was a story about Donald taking one of the electric vans used by the porters in the grounds of the hospital when it was left unattended, driving it around for a distance until he crashed it. A colleague who was enjoying a meal in a restaurant described how Donald entered, was welcomed wholeheartedly by the waiters and provided with a full meal without having to pay for it. When he tried to intervene to pay on Donald's behalf, he was assured by the waiters that this was a regular occurrence. They liked his visits and never expected him to pay.

Although his speech was quite indistinct due to a palate defect, people soon learnt that he was very astute. He had an infinite capacity for acquiring things that he wanted in any conceivable circumstance without having to pay for them. For instance, if it was late and he wanted to return home, he would simply walk into the police station where also he was invariably recognised and welcomed and got the police to ring his home for a lift or even have one from the police themselves.

At other times he was spotted begging in the city centre, selling the 'Big Issue' or putting lots of money into the slot machines in one of the arcades.

He was loved by everyone because of his eccentric and adventurous ways, however, much worry he caused by his late nights and escapades by rail to other towns, not least by the people who comprised his support team. Although he was not an active or productive member of the community in the conventional sense, everyone agreed that he enriched the lives of all who knew him.

Unfortunately, and entirely unexpectedly, Donald became ill one summer and within a few weeks he died of a heart condition at the age of forty-five. This was a tremendously traumatic experience for his carers, who reacted initially in a variety of ways which betrayed their grief and distress, displaying tearfulness, sorrow, recrimination and anger towards one another and his family, who initially expressed the wish for a quiet funeral for Donald.

However, much they aspire to maintaining a professional distance from the people that they support, it is almost inevitable that carers will be affected by the death of service users. Loyal staff members frequently are involved with individuals for many years. They have helped them through many life events and traumas, such as changes in residence, illness and the loss of friends or family. Service users, lacking any meaningful involvement with their families or the skills to make close friendships often develop close relationships with their carers which are reciprocated. When service users do die, staff may need to focus on the needs of other residents and family members and neglect their own need to manage their grief.

Generally, we know the feelings that we are likely to experience when grieving, but seldom reflect on them and prepared adequately for the process.

Classically the stages of grief are as follows:

1.   Denial and Isolation
The first reaction to someone's death of a cherished loved one is to deny the reality of the situation as a form of defence mechanism that buffers the immediate shock and allows us to cope with the immediate pain of loss.

2.   Anger
Eventually denial cannot be maintained and often is superseded by intense anger aimed at friends or family, inanimate objects, complete strangers, doctors and other health professional who treated the dying person or even the person that we have lost. Rationally, we know the person is not to be blamed but we may resent the person for leaving us. We feel guilty for being angry, and this makes us angrier. We may direct our anger at ourselves because of our perception that we could have done more.

3.   Bargaining
The normal reaction to feelings of helplessness and vulnerability is often a need to regain control –
•   If only we had sought medical attention sooner…
•   If only we got a second opinion from another doctor…
•   If only we had tried to be a better person toward them…

4.   Depression
Initially we might feel depressed about the practicalities relating to the loss. We worry about the costs and burial. We worry that, in our grief, we have spent less time with others that depend on us. This may well be followed by sadness relating to the actual loss of the person.

5.   Acceptance

This phase is marked by withdrawal and calm. We are not happy, but we are learning to accept our loss.

Staff should be educated at least in the stages that have been described above, with the understanding that each individual might experience the stages differently or not the same order that you would expect. They should be given the chance to reflect how they might react when someone that they care for does die.

It is important to acknowledge that people's response to a death might vary widely due to temperament or religious faith. Some people may naturally have a more accepting, resigned approach to any loss, including death, or readily derive consolation from their belief in an afterlife. Older people also may be more inured to the fact that we all pass on eventually whilst a teenager may be quite traumatised by what may be their first experience of death, particularly if it is sudden. Also, individual reactions to the demise of a service user might be affected by an association with a recent personal loss or the anniversary of a family member's death.

Services often use the key worker system where team members take a special interest in specific individuals, ensuring among other things that service users have adequate personal possessions and clothing, that they maintain contact with their families and their special occasions, including birthdays and Christmases, are remembered and celebrated appropriately. A member of staff may fulfil the key worker role for many years and develop a really close bond. When staff provide support to service users through their different life events including their personal losses, illnesses, changes in residence activity, loss of mobility due to age, those experiences can also cause a very close relationship, particularly when service users have limited social support network or little family involvement and appear so reliant on carers for their physical and emotional needs. In these circumstances, the loss of the person with a learning disability has infinitely more impact than the death of someone with whom one has a more traditional staff/client relationship.

The great temptation that carers are subjected to is to simply carry on as if nothing has happened in a misguided belief that this reaction what is expected of them and is the right and proper 'professional' response. Immediately following a death, all the circumstances conspire towards steering them down the road to this approach. Straightaway there are practical things to do like ensuring the body is presented in a respectful manner, summoning GPs to certify death, liaison with hospital staff if that is where the death has occurred, relatives, colleagues and other service users to be informed in a tactful compassionate manner. Then funeral arrangements have to be made, sometimes with staff having to take the lead if there is no family involvement or a degree of negotiation undertaken with relatives, either to assert the last wishes of the deceased person or ensure a consensus about the exact nature of the funeral service. Finances have to be put in order and possessions disposed of, even though this might be quite harrowing for staff. Once the funeral is over, there is usually a financial imperative for services to start considering referrals so that the empty space is filled quickly and the process of integrating new residents becomes a consuming focus. Of course, the other service users still have their practical and emotional needs to be met, including support to cope with their own grief.

When a team do experience a death, carers really welcome someone from within the parent organisation, but external to the team at least acknowledging their loss and the variety of emotions people might feel. Team members may feel a variety of emotions, not all of them negative and injurious. They may feel sad, not simply due to loss, but also due to the perception that the person who has died had lead an unfulfilled or even wasted life due a long period of institutionalisation or circumscribed opportunities because of the severity of his or her disability. Staff might feel guilty because they think that they have not done enough for the person immediately prior to death or even blame themselves for its occurrence. They may feel remorse and shame for angry thoughts towards the deceased person or believe that they are at fault for not helping them do more with their life. There may be anger directed at the person who has died for leaving everyone, towards oneself and colleagues or aimed at other services which staff think weren't responsive enough or could have listened to them more or done more to save the person concerned. The Death by Indifference report identifies that the unwarranted death of people with learning disabilities in acute services is a very common event and staff anger against other agencies is consequently highly likely.

Sudden death due to conditions like epilepsy or accidents such as choking, a hazard that people with disabilities are particularly vulnerable to, can be especially traumatic for carers, especially those who are on the scene, are faced with the sudden life threatening crisis and may be put in the position of attempting to revive the dying service user to no avail. One can imagine the extreme emotions that team members would experience in those circumstances, such as self-blame, recrimination, guilt, shock and anxiety and the impact on their general health and normal patterns of living including eating, sleeping and the ability to enjoy activities.

There is no template of support which will suit all teams and individuals. A simple session of debriefing which explores the predominant emotions with at least some of the team may suffice. Sometimes people may need to be facilitated in reflecting on the reasons for the person's death and in making a journey to the point where they realise that in fact there was nothing that any of them could have done to prevent the death. Also, team members may need to have the chance to talk about the deceased person's life, to celebrate the good things that happened and the person's qualities and characteristics, to share anecdotes, and to feel reassured that they had supported the person that they had lost to lead a pleasant and worthwhile life.

If the predominant emotion is anger towards other agencies because of perceived lack of care, the home manager may need support and signposting towards pursuing the matter further either through discussions with clinicians and other health professionals to establish the true nature of the care that the deceased person or through the external agency's complaints procedure.

It is possible that individual members of a team could have different emotions or a combination of them, and it is important that this possibility is acknowledged, and each person receives individualised support if necessary. Some team members may be more vulnerable to becoming distressed by a death because they had a particularly close relationship, they were on duty when the person died or they had had particularly traumatic interactions with external services or relatives. Another factor might be that the death had occurred close to the anniversary of a personal loss or just after a bereavement and may need special care and attention. Home and project managers are a group of people whose needs could be particularly neglected because of their involvement in the practical aspects that need to take place immediately after a death and the need to inform relatives and others and the continuing need to support colleagues and other service users through their loss.

Often a funeral that does justice to the deceased person and that serves as a chance to celebrate his or her life has a therapeutic effect.

Another form of loss which carers can experience is when a service user develops dementia. This seems an especially poignant occurrence when the sufferer has Down syndrome and so starts to decline both mentally and physically at quite a premature age, often in their fifties. The deterioration may be very rapid and cataclysmic, with changes in mood and mental ability matched by the loss of self-help skills, such as the ability to feed and dress oneself or the onset of incontinence and loss of mobility. Carers may feel that they have lost everything about that person which made them special and individual and mourn the loss of ability and dignity that the person endures. They may well go through all the stages of grief associated with death, including denial, intense sadness and anger directed at the disabled person or at themselves for feeling that way. Also, they can experience frustration and irritability because the person that they have known and liked for many years is so changed and may have become lethargic, stubborn or bad tempered. It is not unusual for someone with Downs syndrome to develop unsociable habits in the early stages of dementia, such urinating or stripping off in inappropriate places, or to become confused as to what time of day it is and do things like getting undressed and ready for bed at unusual times. Their uncertainty and anxiety might make them clingy and want to be around their staff members all the time. They may ask the same question over and over again due to short term memory loss or the need for reassurance because of their insight into how they are changing.

Also, carers often want to do all that they can to ensure that the service user who is developing dementia remains in their own home and continues to pursue all their interests as long as possible. However, they may be troubled by the prospect of their client physically deteriorating so much that the property that has been home for many years is no longer suitable. They possibly will doubt that they have the necessary skills to support someone who has become completely physically dependent and a wheelchair user.

Teams would benefit from a chance to explore the likely progress and outcome of someone who has started to suffer from dementia, both to gain an appreciation that deterioration may be quite slow although virtually inevitable but also to understand fully how physically and intellectually disabled the person that they support might eventually become.

Armed with that knowledge, they can readily grasp that in fact the service user is not going to change out of all recognition in the short term. This is helpful in overcoming those feelings of sadness associated with what appear to be the impending loss of the person's essential nature.

Also, staff will have a more realistic understanding of the challenge ahead of them, that significant deterioration is inevitable and are able to start preparing themselves emotionally for the changes to come in the service user so that they are better able to cope with their psychological impact.

One of the difficulties inherent in this sort of scenario is that it is not possible to predict either the rate or the particular form that the decline in skills, behaviour or mental functioning might take. As such, team members will always have that sense of uncertainty about how things might progress. Sometimes people with Downs syndrome might become more aggressive or alternatively lethargic and unmotivated. They may lose skills at different rates and in a different order compared to others with the same condition. Ultimately one would expect that eventually the service user experiencing Alzheimer's disease would become incontinent, lose the ability to dress and feed themselves, lose the capacity to walk and become immobile and apparently have very little awareness of his or her surroundings or recognise anybody. However, the rate and speed of deterioration varies so much from individual to individual and, although likely, is not inevitable.

Nevertheless, it is still beneficial good that carers learn the full extent and range of deterioration the service users may experience. This enables them to develop a heightened perception of the many aspects of potential deterioration and more readily spot early signs of decline in a particular area. As such carers would be more able to respond to and accommodate those changes.

Also, staff can start thinking about the areas of development that they might need to address if they wish to achieve the usual aim to which people aspire, namely helping the service user to live in his/her cherished home, especially as carers readily appreciate that remaining in a familiar setting has great benefits for people who are losing skills and cognitive ability.

The main purpose of carers learning which changes in the environment and approaches would be beneficial for someone who is developing dementia is of course to support that person in the most effective way. However, team members derive great comfort from knowing that they can proactively do things that will help to mitigate the service user's loss of skills and mental ability and maintain quality of life. They are less likely to feel disempowered and anxious about meeting the challenge of supporting someone who is undergoing such profound physical and mental changes.

There are several scenarios which may lead to an individual with learning disabilities having to leave the services that they have lived in for many years. They may have become too frail or limited in mobility to be accommodated in a conventional house. Their behaviour might have become too challenging to be managed in the particular settings that they are currently living.

Staff may become uncomfortable and frustrated because they realise that an individual would benefit from a more intensive support service, due to challenging behaviour or needs associated with deterioration in physical or mental health but cannot immediately expedite a change in service for that individual. Conversely, someone may desire a more independent lifestyle that could only be achieved by moving to his or her own accommodation but are hindered in their support of this cause by concerns that social workers or relatives may have about managing the risk.

It is likely that carers will experience a whole range of emotions in these circumstances compounded by their perception that they have a disproportionately greater impact on the lives of service users with severe and profound disabilities or on the autistic spectrum who are likely to have very limited networks of support.

In an article in which he focuses on staff attributions and emotional responses to challenging behaviour, Cudre-Mauroux (2010) articulates that staff may blame themselves for the appearance of such behaviour because they perceive themselves to be negligent, or they may feel ashamed because they think their lack of ability has contributed to extreme expressions of distress in people that they have supported devotedly. They may also feel despair because those types of behaviour appear so intractable and unsusceptible to any form of treatment or amelioration.

I would contend that carers feel similar emotions for a whole range of adverse situations that occur in the lives of people with learning disabilities. They could become annoyed, piteous, despondent, frustrated, feel powerless and blame themselves in trying to manage any of the scenarios necessitating the changes described above.

In all of these circumstances, carers would benefit from a full understanding of the nature of the conditions and illnesses that a service user is experiencing, and a realistic appreciation of their likely progression. In this way they can learn what type of service is needed for a particular individual. As in many circumstances, what is helpful for the client benefits the people that are supporting him or her. The adaptations to the home environment, referrals for multidisciplinary support, acquisition of aids and specialised equipment, applications for funding to provide more support hours have the main benefit of maximising the likelihood that people remain living in their homes and also reassure staff that they are doing everything in their power to prevent the necessity for a potentially demoralising move.

If someone does have to transfer to another service, carers derive tremendous comfort from knowing that a process has been followed which totally focuses on the needs of that individual, rather than one which is driven by the wishes of others, and the pressures experienced by social workers and commissioners.

Team members like to be involved in exploring options for the people they support and through fulfilling this role derive reassurance that service users have a choice in where they will live in the future, are going to places which can cope with their needs and have a compassionate, progressive ethos. Similarly, they have a place in supporting those who wish to lead a more independent lifestyle, acting as advocates on their behalf in an assertive manner. By overcoming opposition from family members or barriers erected by those who should be using their professional position to seek more appropriate services, carers may secure their own peace of mind whilst ensuring that the wishes of service users are fully respected.

When a transition proves to be inevitable, it may not have the same impact as someone dying. It will nevertheless affect carers. The impact of such transitions may be eased by carers having the opportunity to talk about their emotions without fear of judgement or ridicule, either at team meetings, during one to one supervisions or in informal contexts, especially at crucial point of a transition.

Chapter 5
The Needs of Home and Project Managers

For many years it has been acknowledged by senior managers, other practitioners, colleagues, the academic community (Elliott and Rose, 1997; Rose and others, 2000) and by the group in question that managers for homes and projects which provide services for people with learning disabilities are subjected to a high level of stress as they seek to fulfil their role.

Increasingly residential homes provide services for people who have a high level of needs as the provision of support for more able people becomes more individualised and reflects their greater capacity for independence with the growth of accommodation in supported living contexts. This concentration of needs, whether related to emotional fragility, poor mental health, sensory and mobility deficits or the multiplicity of health concerns experienced by people with profound disabilities impacts on all direct care staff. However, the home manager, as the person ultimately held accountable for the provision of care in the eyes of CQC, parent organisations family members, associated professionals and every other stakeholder, assumes the major burden of tension and anxiety attendant on this responsibility.

Home and project managers fulfil their duties in a very public arena. CQC reports, which may expose flaws in services, are published on the internet and can be read by any member of the public. Inspections occur each year and are nerve racking. An organisation may impose a system of regular internal inspection, intended to be helpful in revealing failings that can be speedily addressed in anticipation of the dreaded statutory inspection, but also potentially distressful.

Other agencies, internal or external may annually examine specific aspects of the home, such as health and safety assessors, environmental health inspectors or financial auditors, with the expectation that the manager will be present for their visits and provide a prompt response to their findings and requirements, including action planning to address any problems.

The general experience for managers is that they potentially can feel overwhelmed by the numerous inspections that occur and by the obligation to swiftly deal with matters that arise, especially as the identification of failings can be demoralising and stigmatising.

Added to that, especially with the rise in the use of emails as a form of communication, managers frequently perceive that they are assailed by many requests for information and responses to be provided within unrealistic timescales concerning matters that they regard as at least non-urgent or even completely trivial. Managers feel that there is often a lack of understanding amongst those who have never worked in care settings of the many functions that they typically have to perform and the disjointed nature of manager's working days.

Sometimes correspondents have fully mastered the etiquette of email communication and give the impression of being confrontational or insensitive. For instance, excessive use of capitals in emails can be interpreted as being intimidatory and disquieting. Also, telephone communications from other agencies or family members can be mildly upsetting for managers by virtue of an abruptness of tone or insistence on an immediate response on the part of the telephone caller. Of course, any member of the team can be subjected to this. However, the home manager is much more likely to deal with phone calls of a controversial nature or from people requiring a swift response to their demands.

These occurrences seem minor and inconsequential. Nevertheless, the intrusion of such negative interactions is interspersed with all the other tasks and duties that a home manager has to undertake during an average day. The job of a home manager is testing in terms of the variety of roles and approaches that they need to assume. During the span of one working day, it is conceivable that he or she might support service users in routine aspects of care or intervene in a situation of behaviour disturbance, answer the phone to relatives, senior managers or external agencies, sometimes to deal with controversial issues, give one to one supervision sessions to a junior employee, teach a student nurse, or tackle disciplinary and development needs, whilst attempting to do essential administrative tasks like preparing duty sheets or complete financial documentation.

Unforeseen circumstances like staffing shortages, health emergencies safeguarding instances may entirely cut across the plans that managers make and cause them to shelve tasks which, although may not be urgent, are important and necessary to maintain standards, such providing supervision sessions and updating Essential Lifestyle Plans. This leads to feelings that one is always reacting to emergencies all the time, can never get on top of his or her workload and is forever neglecting aspects of work directly related to service user care.

The most debilitating aspect of home managers role may well be the range of different emotions and approaches experienced and adopted some days as a typical leader shifts from sometimes consoling staff, being conciliatory and facilitative and then highly directive and assertive depending on the exigencies of the day. These changes in management style might be accompanied feelings of sadness, self recrimination and guilt due to sympathy with staff that have undergone stressful or anger and reproach towards team members because of their mistakes or deficiencies in their practice. The intensity of emotions may be exacerbated by the close relationship managers have with their junior staff that have worked loyally for them and been supportive when they, the managers, have had difficulties.

Of course, when something very serious occurs, such as the death of a service user or an abusive incident, home managers feel the same anguish as the rest of the team. However, they usually choose to suppress feelings of grief and emotional pain and avoid an outward display in order to be a more effective support to distressed team members, a strategy which facilitates the processing of emotions for junior carers but means that managers do not always effectively deal with their own feelings.

During altercations with visiting professionals and family members, it is inevitable that managers will take a lead in those interactions, and endure the bulk of the negative upsetting criticism that might be expressed, leading again to feelings of anger or self-blame which have to be kept in check as they seek to maintain a professional, empathic and problem solving demeanour.

Rose and others (2000) and Elliott and Rose (1997) confirmed to a degree in their research findings that home managers, although perhaps stimulated by the variety of their roles, are exposed to more stressors than their colleagues and so have a greater chance of experiencing anxiety. They suggest that, although home managers often succeed in protecting their team members from stress, the reciprocal relationship is not as effective, i.e. due to the intrinsic nature of that relationship, direct care staff cannot offer the same degree of support to managers. Managers often have been promoted from the staff team and are viewed differently by their colleagues because the former need to sometimes make unpopular decisions or reprimand staff.

Home managers are based on the same site as the team and so have much greater opportunity to offer both formal and ad hoc support to their junior staff, whereas their line managers are usually a geographically and psychologically distant presence and so can only provide peripheral supervision.

In the studies referred to the size of a team was regarded as significant. A big team would appear to suggest an enhanced support network. However, the larger the number of care workers a home manager has to lead, the higher the propensity for stress because of the need to provide a greater degree of supervision.

Home managers also were found to act as mediators between the team and the demands of the organisation, a function which impacted on managers' tension levels. Role ambiguity, in the form of conflict between the administrative and caring facets of a home manager's workload, was identified as another significant stressor.

Often home managers will cover absences which arise at short notice either for budgetary reasons, to save booking expensive agency staff, or simply because there is no-one else available. Inevitably this course of action increases their workload or means that time allocated for necessary administrative tasks is used for directly supporting service users.

Working extra shifts unexpectedly also can impair home managers' relationships with their families, which may already be strained due to the need to work 'unsocial hours' and the impact on managers' moods due to the emotional demands of leading care services.

Generally, home and project managers may increasingly experience a blurring of the delineations between personal and work life, especially if they are regularly contacted by team members for advice and help when they are not 'on duty'.

The role of home and project managers consists of a high degree of responsibility which cannot be avoided. It is an inherent part of the occupation, enshrined in the job description and accepted and understood by those appointed the position. Nevertheless, it appears that they are subjected to an array of stressors not readily appreciated by line managers or outside agencies and sometimes by the managers themselves. Often, they are drawn into complex and emotionally demanding relationships with colleagues, service users and family members resulting in an incremental erosion of their personal time and boundaries between home and work life.

Notwithstanding the inevitable demands and responsibilities of the managerial role in care services, there are strategies that can be adopted to mitigate the effect of the stressors that I have described.

For instance, home managers can adopt a management style which encourages initiative and embracing responsibility within the team. If carers are allowed to develop a degree of autonomy, they are more readily able to assume tasks delegated by home/project managers and take on a greater sense of ownership within the team, more readily accepting responsibility for supporting one another rather than feeling that they need to go to the manager with every problem.

Of course, embracing this particular managerial style, often termed 'Theory Y' from the works by McGregor (1960) has its perils. Sometimes trusting staff and relinquishing control of some aspects of the work environments can result in carers making mistakes, which the manager has to rectify. However, team members who feel empowered have been developed so that they have the capacity to deal with sensitive and exceptional circumstances and have acquired the confidence to act autonomously. They are more likely to act with greater efficiency in a variety of scenarios. This can have beneficial consequences as home managers are less likely to be contacted 'out of hours' for every problem that arises and no longer become the sole focus for problem solving and provision of support on a day to day basis.

Sanderson (2003) talks about the development of 'person-centred teams' comprising of people who can act independently, with a degree of initiative and are self-reliant.

It is also helpful if senior managers and administrative staff have a degree of empathic insight into the demands of the home manager's role so that they are less likely to make requests for action and information within timescales which are unreasonable and unrealistic. Senior managers who have had the experience of being a home manager will have acquired greater comprehension about issues which affect the well-being of home and project managers, but that in itself is no guarantee of an understanding of their stressors. Also, such attitudes can be inculcated through senior managers actually spending more time in residential settings and using one to one sessions as a medium for the supervisee to disclose, without fear and recrimination, tensions and anxieties and seek help in resolving difficulties. Ideally, supervision sessions should be used for that purpose and not solely for the business-like discussion of actions and outcomes. However, home managers may prefer not to reveal too much about what they may regard as their weaknesses for fear that they will be regarded by others as inadequate and incapable of doing their job effectively.

The onus is on senior managers to recognise this and build a relationship of trust and positive regard towards residential and project managers. Of course, senior managers are appointed to ensure that their subordinates do their jobs properly and sometimes have to reprimand or even discipline them. However, the starting point in the relationship should be one of mutual respect and acknowledgement of the difficulties that home managers encounter on a daily basis, without seeking to apportion blame and criticise too readily.

This attitude should be adopted by senior managers when they perform internal audits of services. Home managers can easily become oppressed by the amount of scrutiny that their areas of work receive. Visits from external agencies such as CQC, environmental health and independent financial auditors are always going to be the most arduous of these inspections because of their extra level of formality and legal status. However, an organisation may choose to do regular internal reviews of a variety of aspects within a residential setting or supported living project. Areas that are checked might include care planning, statutory documentation, the administration of health and safety issues and local financial procedure.

Locality and area managers, health and safety, financial and other specialised auditors should perform these organisational inspections in a manner which is facilitative rather than castigatory. They should regard the process as an opportunity to identify deficits in services in a less punitive way than is the case when external, statutory agencies inspect. Notice should be given for each inspection and clear guidance on the areas that are to be examined. The audit should be performed in a way which is does not add to the home manager's stress levels even if there issues which need to be promptly addressed. The auditor should negotiate reasonable time scales for action planning and dealing with service deficiencies and offer help to achieve those action points. For instance, the person doing the internal inspection may know of peers who have formats and systems that they can share with their home manager colleagues or be able to offer specific help themselves. The internal audit process should be regarded as much as an educative process which, as well as helping home mangers to achieve statutory requirements and to increase standards, aids them to navigate the formal inspections with confidence and preparedness.

A CQC inspection ranks as one of the more stressful aspects of a home manager's job role, by virtue of the oppressive nature that such intense scrutiny and also the inevitable action planning required to address compliance issues. It is neither possible nor desirable for home managers to be 'on call' and attend work for every serious exigency, including CQC inspections. Therefore, it is important that team members are prepared for this process so that they can effectively communicate to a CQC inspector and respond professionally to the latter's queries and requests to look at documentation. Areas where very specific and focussed preparation might be given include information concerning CQC standards, the actual areas that the inspector is there to assess, safeguarding matters and reporting procedures, knowledge of the Mental Capacity Act and Deprivation of Liberty Safeguards and simply knowing where relevant documentation is kept.

Junior staff being able to cope with unannounced inspections in a confident, assertive and capable manner can be very reassuring and stress relieving for home and project managers who feel less that they have to be on the premises to deal with every sensitive or controversial event.

Generally, managers should aspire to share the burden of responsibility by involving team members as much as possible in fulfilling administrative tasks like monitoring health and safety standards or completing financial returns.

Aside from task orientated delegation it is good for Mangers to become aware of the general qualities of team members so that they have a more sophisticated appreciation of how individuals can contribute and match tasks or roles more effectively to their colleagues. Belbin (2010) identified nine team member roles:

1. The plant (someone who revels in solving difficult problems)
2. Resource manager (good at exploring potentiality for resources and making external contacts)
3. Co-ordinator (the person who brings everyone together and values them all for their different skills)
4. Shaper (focuses on setting of objectives and priorities and imposing some shape and pattern to group discussions)
5. Monitor/ evaluator (analyses problems, evaluates ideas and suggestions)
6. Team worker (good at improving communication and nurturing team spirit)
7. Implementer (good at actually putting plans into action)
8. Completer (applies great attention to detail and maintains a sense of urgency)
9. Specialist (has a distinct body of knowledge or level of expertise essential to the achievement of objectives)

Developing an understanding of how team members fit these various roles can be a help in guiding a manager, not only to match tasks and roles with particular individuals, but also to avoid allocating jobs or functions which that person is not temperamentally suitable to execute. Also, informed by knowledge of the 'Belbin' roles, managers are more likely to cultivate a greater appreciation of their own strengths and aptitudes and the areas where they should delegate to colleagues who are more effective than them in a particular role.

Other models of personality and learning styles which can enhance managers' perspectives of their strengths and support needs include the work of Myers and Briggs (2010), which delineates psychological types in terms of the combinations between extraversion, introversion, intuition and sensing, and Honey and Mumford's (1989) work on activists, pragmatists, reflectors and theorists.

Managers often complain that they simply do not have enough time to complete all the tasks that either their managers or they themselves expect them to achieve. Also, the role of home or project manager can become quite disjointed during some days with unexpected exigencies, interruptions and crises cutting right across what they originally had planned. Frequently they will adopt the coping strategy of taking work home (e.g compiling the staff duty sheet) and complete it there, or simply extend their length of time at work with no likelihood of reclaiming the time owed to them. One of my 'strategies' as when I was a home manager was to work extra shifts as a support worker, when there were gaps in the duty sheet, to give me more hours to fulfil my management tasks. In fact, the outcome was usually increased stress for me as the process of juggling administrative tasks with service user support needs caused me tensions related to role stress.

Teaching time management techniques is no panacea, but surely must be a help. These could include simple strategies:

> such as building of an awareness of the time that they have available;
> developing an understanding of their priorities, planning according to those priorities;

> conscious allocation of slots for tasks allocating sufficient time to complete what they wish to do, and so avoiding time lost through having to constantly pick up the threads of a task when it is started again;
> Learning to be definite in managing interruptions and effective delegation.

The latter has its perils. One should never delegate tasks which are sensitive, controversial or beyond the abilities or experience of the person who has been asked to complete them. However, delegation should be a constant way of life for managers; they should actively seek to hand over as many tasks as possible to junior staff both to relieve their own workload and to give opportunities for employees to develop and extend their perspective of their roles. Specifically, by ensuring that they receive focussed admin support, managers can off load time consuming administrative tasks such as resolution of financial records and transactions or ordering supplies, to members of staff who have been trained to do such duties speedily and efficiently.

Also, managers often find it difficult to say 'no' and end up assuming duties and tasks which are burdensome. Sometimes they might find themselves intimidated by the demands and opinions of external professionals, members of their own team, external employees of their own organisation or service user family members. It is easy to respond in a way that is highly defensive and aggressive or overly compliant with the wishes of others. Moreover, they may have tricky encounters and communications with immediate superiors and their own team members around unreasonable demands and performance or disciplinary issues which are made more difficult by the closeness of their relationships.

Many managers, although capable, experienced and knowledgeable, have not fully developed their powers of assertion and so may require specific training in this area. This may include learning about the different Life Positions that can be adopted:

Passive behaviour (I'm not OK – You're OK)
Manipulative behaviour (I'm not OK – You're not OK)
Aggressive behaviour (I'm OK – You're not OK)
Assertive behaviour (I'm OK – You're OK)

Home and project managers are often notorious for attending assiduously to the support needs of their staff whilst neglecting their own. They should be encouraged to develop an awareness of their own support needs and how they can be met. It may well be that very specific elements of a job are more stressful for individuals. For some, speaking in meetings might be their most onerous task, others find routine completion of paperwork a chore whilst liaising with family members about contentious topics is most stressful for another group. Being honest about and acknowledging one's areas of vulnerability is the starting point for addressing them. Practical support can be given to help individuals develop and cope with the area of work that cause them the most anxiety in the form of specific tuition in talking to groups, conflict management training, and practical tips from other home managers about documentation.

One of the barriers for home managers is acknowledging that there is actually a problem which has a set of solutions. Often managers will soldier on, accepting that high levels of tension and anxiety are their inevitable lot and taking few steps to deal with their situation. Sometimes they are not even aware of the levels of tension.

Very little attention has been given over the years to teaching managers relaxation techniques, ways to cope with stress actually whilst at work and to off load it once the working day is finished. It is often tempting for managers to resort to traditional but not necessarily effective ways to relieve tension, including drinking lots of alcohol, smoking and other forms of recreational drug use or overeating. In truth different personalities cope with stress in very diverse ways. One person might prefer to unwind by participating in some form of exercise, another by pursuing more sedate hobbies;

for someone else an evening at the pub or a night spent at a club are more effective stress relievers.

Given that we are all different and have widely varying approaches to relaxation, it is important that managers reflect on their stress levels, find ways to monitor them and learn which relaxation strategies suit them best. It should be standard practice that people attend workshops which present to them and allow them to try out a variety of relaxation techniques. The content of these sessions might include education on quite mundane subjects like the importance of eating and drinking adequately during the working day, deep breathing exercises or progressive muscle relaxation. It also might include exploration of more esoteric methods such as positive imagery, meditation and Cognitive Behaviour Therapy techniques, including 'mindfulness'.

Alan's story (how specific education in relaxation techniques can benefit an individual)

My final home manger post was as the leader of a team which supported a group of men who had severe complex emotional needs related to conditions like autism, Fragile X and epilepsy. There was great potentiality for aggression occurring which the staff largely averted due to a good understanding of their service users and a proactive approach. However, this process of constant vigilance with regard to individual triggers, early warning signs and swift intervention brought its own set of tensions. I arranged for the team to attend a stress management workshop facilitated by a colleague, who, to my surprise, started with a lengthy session on the harmful effects of not drinking enough during the working day. I realised that, although better than I was as a young man, my fluid intake each day was still rather low and often consisted of a disproportionate amount of coffee, making me more likely to be irritable. When the workshop was concluded, I made a resolution to drink at least 2 litres of squash and cut down my consumption of coffee to three cups a day.

In a subsequent session, I also learnt the usefulness of the technique 'mindfulness' as a way to switch off at regular intervals during the day even if only for a minute or so and to deter me from racing from one task to another without taking pause to think and relax for even a second.

Sadie and Terry's stories (How particular developmental needs can be addressed using external or internal resources tailored to individual needs)

Along with several other managerial colleagues, Sadie disclosed to her area manager that she had an anxiety about speaking in groups at formal meetings particularly. Her organisation arranged for her and her associates to undergo a training course comprising four evening sessions spread over four weeks and lead by an expert in this subject. The course gave her opportunity to practice public speaking in a safe environment and offered her practical suggestions about how she could cope when having to perform this aspect of her role. Although she felt nervous attending the course and hasn't had her anxiety totally allayed, she feels better about speaking to groups than was previously the case.

When I visited Terry's residential home for a regular internal audit using a format based on CQC standards, although many of the areas that I examined were entirely satisfactory, there was a particular area of documentation relating to service user Health Action Plans that needed improvement. I was able to suggest that Terry seek advice from a home manager colleague who I knew from auditing her home had constructed excellent Health Action Plans. Terry was able to view how her team had used the HAP format and was able update those for which he was responsible much more quickly than if he was 'starting from scratch'.

It is important that home managers are given prompt training as a group on specific areas relating to their role so that they can action plan to accommodate any changes in practice and also derive peer support more readily, using training sessions for discussion and problem solving.

Commonly, home and project managers can feel very isolated and not have many opportunities to receive support from colleagues who are in similar positions. They are frequently 'reinventing the wheel' in settings geographically remote from one another rather than having the chance to learn from one another's experiences, successes and mistakes. Organisations frequently hold home and project manager meetings but for an entirely different function, namely the dissemination of information relevant to services and to discuss administrative matters. Managers would probably benefit more from opportunities to meet as a group to share concerns and find solutions to difficulties actually within services.

There are many demands on home mangers to ensure that documentation is maintained to a high standard due to legal, organisational, professional and ethical reasons. Also, documentation has to be accessible to service users requiring the use of graphics and photographs. It is not possible for one person to maintain standards in this area and all staff should receive IT training or literacy development so that the burden is shared. The creation of professional and accessible documents requires very specific skills and the judicious use of administrative support can be a great help to home and project managers.

One of the areas where home and project managers often struggle is setting a limit on communication and involvement with their work place. The onset of communication by emails whilst beneficial for their speed and immediacy is injurious because there is a constant temptation to access work messages from home. I have colleagues who habitually check their work email account first thing in the morning at seven am and again, late in the evening, or will look at them on their days off, including weekends. Such practices are highly understandable as managers seek to keep on top of their work load and anticipate problems before they go actually go into the work setting. However, it feels that whatever the time constraints and responsibilities, allowing work matters to intrude into personal lives is injurious, particularly when some of the problems, such as safeguarding issues and service user illness may be laden with emotional stress.

Chapter 6
Managing Relationships with Family Members and Other Professionals

Those unfortunate people who were coerced into living in long stay hospitals throughout the earlier part of the twentieth century commonly lost touch with their families. In the early years of my career, I met many who had had that experience, including a man who, at the age of four, came to live in a Bristol 'colony', but originated from a completely different part of the country. We can infer that the stigma associated with 'mental deficiency', poverty and the lack of social mobility that appertained in the 1920s and '30s conspired to ensure that this man and many others completely lost touch with their parents, siblings and extended families. Residents of long stay hospitals often lived well into old age and died without ever renewing contact their relatives.

Even if parents aspired to visiting their children in such institutions, barriers were put in the way by the hospital administrative staff; they could not visit in a spontaneous way, but instead had to make appointments to visit and no private areas were made available for visits in establishment which were grim and unwelcoming. Hospitals usually were situated in semi rural areas which had limited access to public transport. Sometimes parents of children newly admitted were told not to visit for a few weeks to allow them to 'settle in', irrespective of how young the children were and the severity of their disability or sensory impairment.

There is still a possibility that young people especially can have their family ties ruptured temporarily due to placements in residential schools and colleges or because of admission to treatment centres and medium secure facilities not necessarily located in the person's place of origin. Notwithstanding, most people with learning disabilities grow up as an integral and loved part of their families and maintain contact with parents, brothers and sisters throughout their lives.

The value of the input and support provided by families is now fully acknowledged and appreciated; parents and other close relatives are regarded as an essential part of the network available to those who have learning disabilities. They are welcomed as visitors in homes and projects, encouraged to contribute to Person Centred Planning, act as advocates, give support during medical appointments and maintain social contact. The moral rights that families have to play a full part in the lives of people with disabilities and the value of those relationships are indisputable.

Nevertheless, there is much scope for dispute and conflict between family members and residential or supported living staff. It is not always the case that parental or sibling contact is altruistic or entirely benign. Sometimes family members seek to exploit their disabled relatives for financial gain or there may be concerns about physical or sexual exploitation. A common of area of disquiet relates the management of benefits; parents may have become used to receiving benefits on behalf of their disabled children and coming to rely on it as an element of their total family income rather than keeping it separate for the use by the individuals for whom it is exclusively intended. When there is a change of circumstances such as the person with learning disabilities entering residential care, tensions may arise when the parents continue to act as appointees and do not make such benefits available for their children. If this state of affairs persists, it may be deemed to be abusive and require a safeguarding alert, a process in which care and support staff may become implicated, impairing relationships with family members.

Sometimes care staff and parents, in particular, may have significant differences of opinion about the level of risk that someone with a learning disability should be exposed to. The former, understandably, may have a more protective attitude towards their children than paid carers which can place the latter in a difficult position, especially if it is service users themselves who wish to try new and potentially risky activities.

Occasionally, family members might have limited self-awareness of the impact of their approach towards their disabled relatives. For instance, they may not fully understand that someone who has autism does not want to be crowded, nagged or fussed over and intrude on his or her personal space excessively.

Some parents hold extremely strong opinions and, notwithstanding the fact that they are now adults, rather dominate their disabled children, take over their meetings and express views which are contrary to the wishes of service users. Their outlook may be rooted in relationship of dependence, which was formerly the case, but fails to acknowledge the development that their children have made or that the latter have changed their interests. For instance, parents might be adamant that their children should continue to go swimming each week because that was a favoured activity when they lived together, without understanding that, in common with the general population, people with learning disabilities alter their preferences and become interested in other things as they grow up.

When relatives sometimes hijack discussions regarding their children and impose their own opinions, even in their presence, there is a clear obligation for carers to assert the rights of service users to be supported in a way which their ideas and wishes take absolute priority. This is a very difficult position to have to adopt because it may lead to acrimony between relatives and carers and feelings of anxiety on the part of clients who feel they are defying their parents or siblings by declaring their own preferences.

Many parents are very knowledgeable about the medical conditions that their children have. It is not inevitable though they will have continually updated their learning and also their perspective on the nature of their children's illnesses may be fixed at the point when they shared a home. For example, they may think that the pattern of their children's epilepsy and the nature of their seizures is the same as formerly when in fact alterations in treatment and lifestyle have caused changes for good or ill.

Most parents have an entirely compassionate and understanding regard for their children. Sometimes though, perhaps because of the burden of caring for difficult people over many years, they may advise staff to take a confrontational and punitive approach to their children if they 'misbehave', advising shouting at them or withholding activities and possessions. Other examples in my experience where family may advocate a more robust approach than would be ethical include tooth brushing or encouraging staff to virtually force their children to go to specific activities. Sometimes quite junior team members are placed in the position of having to refute such approaches and explain the moral and pragmatic reasons why they cannot follow such aversive and abusive courses of action.

Occasionally carers are subjected to strong criticism from relatives, sometimes expressed in a manner that is really impolite and inconsiderate, an experience that can be stressful. Irrespective of whether the criticism is justified or not, encounters of this sort can leave staff feeling vulnerable and demoralised, especially if they occur at times when managers are not readily available for advice and support.

Frequent visitors to homes and projects may, unwittingly or otherwise, develop an inappropriate degree of interest in the affairs of other residents and place members of staff in a difficult position where they have to tactfully deal with attempts to garner information which those visitors have no right to know.

Jane's story

Jane's son, Ian, as well as having a severe intellectual impairment, had autism and severe epilepsy. These conditions often caused him to be often irritable and quite aggressive to other people. His epilepsy, in particular, necessitated him attending appointments at the local hospital with his consultant neurologist every three months. Jane wanted to attend each appointment that Ian had, but was always anxious prior to their occurrence. His care team found her anxiety difficult to cope with particularly because Ian himself became very anxious on these occasions and this was a likely cause of him hitting out at his escorts which was stressful enough in itself. The impact of Jane's anxiety was compounded by her failure to recognise that her habits of fussing around Ian and encroaching on his personal space were also precipitants for his aggression, putting his escorts at risk and possibly jeopardising the success of the appointment.

As can be imagined, it was quite likely that staff would resent her presence regarding her as a hindrance whilst they were trying to do their job and increasing the possibility that they would get hurt. There was another stressor as Jane usually had a different perspective to the staff regarding the impact of his illness and tended to assume that it was worse than clinical records suggested, leading to the possibility of conflicting information being given to his consultant.

It was important that Jane was able to attend the appointments without affecting Ian's anxiety levels and there was an agreement reached regarding the current picture of his medical condition both for Ian's sake and the welfare of his carers.

Careful planning was always needed to ensure that the timing of his arrival at the outpatients department ensured that he did not have to wait too long in the waiting area and it was essential that Jane was involved in that planning, so she was clear about the sequence of actions that were entailed for each appointment and when they would happen.

A senior manager took the lead both in this process and also in meeting with her prior to setting off for the appointment so that a consensus could be attained between care staff and Jane about their views of the current state of Ian's epilepsy.

Ian normally had two supporting staff for any visit to community settings. A third person, almost invariably home or deputy home manager, also attended on these occasions *principally to support Jane and ensure that the correct information was communicated to his consultant.*

Careful planning, extra support and leadership from managers all combined to make these events successful and to minimise the level of stress endured by his staff escorts.

What can help carers to cope with all these potential stressors relating to interactions with family members? A good starting point is to have a staff culture, established by managers, which acknowledges the central role of parents and other close relations in the lives of service users. Staff should be encouraged to embrace suggestions that family members make and any involvement they wish to have. Adopting such a positive attitude from the outset means that carers are not thinking in defensive terms and will greet people in a confident and welcoming manner. This will be noticed by visitors who consequently will be more likely to build warm relationships with staff and seek to work collaboratively.

When disabled people have left the family home and live in residential homes or supported living projects, parents may feel that they now have a diminished role in their children's lives, may worry about the safety of the safety of the latter, feel guilty about no longer being able look after their children anymore and be concerned about leaving them in the care of people that they know little about, particularly in light of recent well publicised incidents of abuse in residential care. It is really important that staff are encouraged to develop empathy about how family members may be feeling. Managers should not assume that support workers will automatically reflect on all the feelings that parents may undergo and the empathy nurturing process may need to be inculcated in a very overt, conscious way

Staff may need specific training to achieve this level of ease in communicating with the relations of service users. They may require help in order to reflect on the limited network of friendships and acquaintances that people with learning disabilities frequently have, resulting in a greater reliance on the support of close family members. They may need to develop and understanding of the reasons for this phenomenon, appreciate how readily disabled people lose contact with childhood friends, have less opportunities to make friendships in valued settings such as work and education, and may well be hampered by severe communication deficits or problems in forming relationships, rooted in difficulties associated with conditions like autism or Fragile X.

Similarly, staff may need facilitation to appreciate the experiences and emotions undergone and felt by parents, that they may have had to battle to secure services, manage the tensions between siblings, ensure that the safety of their disabled children, cope with the anxiety fear and despair associated with challenges and the guilt arising from accepting the need for long term residential care. However, much parents may rationalise that such moves are 'for the best', that young people of all abilities usually leave home at some point, essentially, they are handing over what they see as their family responsibilities to carers that they hardly know, a tremendous leap of faith and trust. If carers become more conscious of these sorts of tensions, it is likely that they will approach family members in a much more empathetic manner and understand better their anxieties and fears.

Not all employees will naturally have a confident and assertive manner towards visitors. It is important that those staff members are given very specific support in the form of training in assertiveness and customer relations, not just as a classroom exercise but also including opportunities to reflect on how they handled situations, facilitated by a mentor who already has a high level of skill in assured communication with family members.

Nevertheless, there may still be occasions when carers have to deal with relatives who express some quite abrasive criticism or robustly assert opinions about possible approaches which are contrary to the wishes of their children, abusive or unethical, or not in the best interests of service users.

In order to help them manage situations like these, knowledge of the same Positive Behavioural Support principles of non-confrontational communication and de-escalation that they have learnt to minimise the impact of challenges from service users are just as applicable when they are faced with verbal aggression from family members. They may well need specific training which helps them identify the key signs present in angry confrontations, irrespective of whether the person is a service user's relative, a visiting professional or a colleague, and how to maintain their composure, stay calm and to manage their words, phrases and body language.

If team members are put in such a position that they have to deal with such scenarios, it is really important that they receive a high degree of managerial support if the family members assertions are unjust, unpleasant and offensive. It may be absolutely appropriate for home mangers to have professional, respectful, courteous, but also very frank conversations with those visitors who are verbally abusive to members of staff.

Occasionally, the things that service users' relatives say can be extremely hurtful, in which case staff should be accorded the same post incident that they would expect if they were subjected to verbal or other challenges form service users. They should not be expected to shrug off such impolite and damaging conversations, but have their feelings acknowledged and respected, given opportunity to have some quiet time away from the client group or opportunities to talk at least briefly about how they feel.

Everything should be done to reassure relatives that care and support are appropriate and compassionate both by prompt discussion of concerns when they are raised, but also by quality audit tools relating to all aspects of care and service user experiences and active formal eliciting of family views.

Many people who have learning disabilities with complex needs require support from a diverse range of specialists from a variety of disciplines, such as psychiatrist, psychologist, speech and language therapists, physiotherapists, behaviour specialist practitioners, epilepsy specialist nurses. In my experience, support staff often lack confidence when they interact with highly educated, confident professional people. They may feel intimidated both when such specialists visit service users in their home and when the support staff are required to attend a multidisciplinary meeting. This may be because they fear criticism of their care and support, feel that they are not articulate enough to express their views or become anxious when they are 'put under the spotlight' and are required to express their views regarding the care of an individual. Perception of the disparity between the level of knowledge and qualification a care worker or personal assistant and professional staff may exacerbate this state of affairs.

Support staff can be helped by general training and guidance on how to express themselves more confidently and assertively. Also, they should be encouraged to prepare for meetings and visits by becoming acquainted with the sort of issues that are likely to be discussed and be able to contribute accurate information and articulate views based on fact rather than ill-informed opinion.

Equally important is the role of training on factors relating to service users' key conditions, such as epilepsy, autism, diabetes, Downs syndrome, Fragile X or whatever else appertains. Armed with such highly specific knowledge and how those factors impact on individuals, support staff are going to be much more confident when asked to contribute to multidisciplinary discussions.

It is vital that support staff learn to appreciate how crucial their perspective is to any such discussions, particularly if those that they support have profound or severe disabilities. They may act as a part of a key working team and in that role and by virtue of their association with service users over the course of many years have become the people who are the most knowledgeable about individuals' needs and mode of communication. An enhanced understanding of the significance of their relationship and knowledge can aid the development of confidence and assertiveness in multidisciplinary discussions.

Chapter 7
The Importance of Personal Characteristics and Values in Carers.
The problem with staff recruitment and retention

On the face of it, it is an obvious point that one of the ways to help employees cope with the stress associated with supporting people with learning disabilities is to appoint the right people in the first place, that is individuals who have the necessary personal qualities, coping skills and temperament for the role as a carer or personal assistant.

As has been noted, what constitutes the key functions and approach of such roles has changed over the years. No longer is it sufficient to provide purely custodial or protective support, carers are now expected to be much more holistic and facilitative in their approach, with the emphasis in encouraging service users to develop, form relationships, engage with the community and become more independent. However, there is a significant body of the caring work force who were appointed when being a support worker was much simpler and simplistic in its scope, who have struggled to adapt to performing the enhanced role described above not because of their incompetence necessarily, but because of lack of clarity regarding the evolution of their function and failure to give adequate support to develop staff. A potential skills deficiency can lead to increased tension as carers struggle to fulfil the more creative and risk-taking aspects of their job.

In such circumstances, it would be unfair to release support workers who have such difficulties unless there was evidence of unwillingness to adapt or overt incompetence. This approach may be emotionally injurious to service users who may have limited social networks but have known those imperfect members of staff for many years, trust them and have a strong emotional attachment to them. Also, losing a significant proportion of the work force would be impracticable. Whatever the state of the current job market and the apparent availability of candidates for prospective vacancies, there is never a guarantee that replacements are going to be more effective or have the stamina for a long-term commitment to supporting this client group. Support for people with learning disabilities remains very labour intensive and nurturing the current work force is a fairer and more realistic strategy than engaging in wishful thinking that they could be replaced by a better one. Person centred approaches and commitment to the belief that people should be given support to develop are fundamental principles that underpin approaches to service users, and it would be a major inconsistency if organisations failed to support their employees to enhance their knowledge skills and attitudes through individualised learning plan.

Notwithstanding the need to return a focus on developing existing staff, a subject that I shall explore later, more attention needs to be applied to the recruitment process, particularly to identifying the qualities and attitudes that are most desirable in prospective carers and personal assistants including those which aid coping with the many stressors that they are likely to encounter.

There has been a shift in recent years towards providing a close match between personal assistants and service users in terms of their mutual interests and hobbies in line with providing support which is highly individualised and as a consequence of increased involvement of clients in recruitment procedures. Although this is a desirable and understandable development, there are concerns that focussing purely on this aspect of abilities is not sufficient and more attention should be given to aspects of personality and core values that prospective candidates may offer.

Research by Rose et al (2003) emphasises the centrality of personality in aiding staff members cope with stress, highlighting the injurious effect of neuroticism and wishful thinking styles of coping; Duran et al (2004) suggest the importance of emotional intelligence in carers, an attribute which incorporates the abilities to attend to, understand, regulate and repair one's emotional states; research commissioned by the MacIntyre care organisation (2011) suggests that, counter to expectations, people who have a greater tendency to introspection, benevolence and empathy are more effective in giving support to those who display problematic, challenging behaviour and evidence greater coping skills. Bill Mumford, the MacIntyre managing director, expressed his initial surprise at the research findings:

'Benevolence and empathy didn't surprise me, but I didn't expect introvert to come up at all. I realised that extroverts don't empower individuals. It made sense that you had to be an introvert because you have to be a good listener. It's about being a person who is more reflective and observational.'

Generally, though, one feels that recruitment in health and social care has tended to attract people who are temperamentally inclined to be activists, who place a high value on 'doing' things and may have a limited approach towards reflection and the more subtle interactions with service users which both decreases their effectiveness and depletes their coping abilities.

Individual personal traits are seen as being highly significant as a predictor of the ability to combat stress. People who have high internal loci of control, who temperamentally regard themselves as being able to influence events, are more likely to exert more effort to change their environment, are better learners and are able to process and use information effectively. These 'hardy' individuals seem also to have an enhanced resistance to stress by virtue of a 'cognitive appraisal system' (Cooper and Bright 2001) comprising three elements:

Commitment, the belief that one's life and activities have meaning and value;

Control, the conviction that one can control events;

Challenge, change in one's life is likely and should be embraced as being beneficial.

Similarly, Kobasa et al (1982) argue some people have a "hardy personality" and felt that those who have a high degree of Hardiness have a strong defence against the negative effects of stress. Key features of this personality also include being high in control, commitment and challenge. Hardy people see themselves as being in control of their lives rather than being controlled by other things have a strong sense of purpose and regard life challenges are seen as something they want to overcome rather than an inevitable cause of stress.

Hardy people have an internal locus of control meaning that they are aware that they cannot influence all the external events that go on in their lives and believe that at in all circumstances, they can choose how they react to stressors and so at the very least have some control over those type of apparently uncontrollable events.

Several instruments have been developed to measure hardiness, the most frequently used being the Personal Views Survey, the Dispositional Resilience Scale and the Cognitive Hardiness Scale. Also, other scales based on hardiness theory have been designed to measure the concept in specific contexts (e.g. parental grief) and populations (e.g. people with chronic illness) suggesting a similar scale could be devised to measure the hardiness of carers.

Conversely, it does seem that a tendency towards neuroticism in a person, with its associated traits of anxiety, depression, moodiness and irritability when confronted with minor obstacles, affects that individual's capacity to deal with stress. It is likely that people affected in this way are more prone to use emotion driven 'wishful thinking' as a coping strategy instead of more effective practical methods; although it is possible also that sometimes this approach is adopted by carers because there are no other coping strategies readily available.

Although some of us have a greater tendency to hardiness it is felt that this personality trait can be developed by teaching people to telling themselves optimistic stories about events in their lives and practise attitudes and techniques like:

> living consciously in the present moment using mindfulness
> promoting self-acceptance and building self-esteem
> being self-responsible for your own feelings rather than surrendering to the whims of others
> developing self-assertiveness where you acknowledge your wants, needs, values, and that it is ok to find appropriate ways to satisfy these
> Practise living purposefully, getting out of hoping and wishing behaviour patterns, and doing what needs to be done to make goals happen
> Practise personal integrity so that your actions reflect your values.
> Spend time relaxing every day
> Learn to regard problems as opportunities, changes as normal, stimulating and inevitable and develop a commitment to a greater, shared purpose.

Belief in control over events in the environment is also associated with better health with respect to diet, potential use of harmful substances and exercise and so development of those traits can help people to adopt a healthier lifestyle, increasing their resilience to stress.

Hardiness can be developed by learning how to regulate your energy and pace yourself in order to sustain the effort needed to deal with stress and strain. This entails developing habits and skills that ensure that people can recover physically, mentally and emotionally from stressful events. The impact of sustained high stress depends on how well you balance the pressures with meeting your recovery needs through relaxation, fun, and play. Loehr (1994) asserts that seeking physical exercise can train the body to have a greater capacity for dealing with stress and the opportunities for employees to follow this course can be facilitated by organisational benefits packages which provide reduced cost Gym Membership or by the encouragement of sports team and exercise clubs in the manner that benevolent employers such as Cadbury's and Fry's pursued in the nineteenth century. Sometimes it seems astonishing that capitalist corporations motivated principally by the desire to make a profit were able to look after their employees more successfully than organisations whose main business is to provide care and support to vulnerable people.

Learning cognitive, behavioural, and interpersonal skills which help carers develop mindfulness techniques, the ability to reflect on events and challenge their own negative assumptions can be beneficial and aid the achievement of an appropriate balance between work, leisure and essential life tasks.

These are some of the techniques that staff could use to develop their 'hardiness:

- ➢ They can learn breathe correctly, usually using their diaphragm, for deep, even breathing.
- ➢ They should foster the habit of relaxing several times during each day
- ➢ Find out which relaxation techniques work for them; this may vary for each individual. Some people play sports whilst others relax in more traditional ways.
- ➢ Try to get into the habit of exercising in a manner which a manner which develops strength, flexibility and aerobic capacity exercises.
- ➢ Learn how to nurture mental toughness and resilience in order to bounce back from setbacks, by fostering a realistic positive attitude.
- ➢ Learn the tricks of managing their time well always including time for themselves, their hobbies and their loved ones.

- Foster an understanding their priorities and goals in life.
- Remember the importance of seek helping from friends or professionals if they feel overwhelmed.
- Realise the importance of accepting life as it is and work with it. They know the difference between acceptance and tolerance and accept others without trying to change them.
- Understand the importance of not holding grudges and striving not to cling on to anger, hostility or aggression
- Learning what constitutes a healthy, moderate and balanced diet suited to their needs and the art of enjoying their food without indulging or binging.
- Cultivate emotional balance. Hardy people may experience extremes of emotions such as sadness, elation or excitement but don't dwell on or remain in those states beyond what you would expect to be the natural time span for their expression.

Several of these ideas are incorporated into the 5 Ways to Wellbeing project commissioned by the government in 2008 and social care organisations should consider educating their staff and encouraging them to follow the following steps to improve their mental and physical wellbeing:

- Connect with others such as family, friends, colleagues, or even new people,

- Be active, try to find a form of exercise that you like

- Keep learning: Sign up for a course, read a book, learn a new skill.

- Give to others: do something nice for a friend or a stranger, volunteer your time or join a community group, give people smiles and thanks.

- Take notice: savour the moment, be aware of what is around you, including what you are feeling

Developing cultures where teams regularly reflect on and celebrate their successes and achievements and develop a shared vision which has the concept of dynamism at its heart. The ability to embrace change is absolutely essential for those who support people with learning disabilities as a major part of their role is to help their client group become more independent, including moving to forms of support which are more individualised and self-directed.

When teams are going through times of change or need to redefine the vision that their service is trying to follow, it may helpful if they engage in generating a SWOT analysis in which they identify their own individual Strengths, Weaknesses, Opportunities and Threats and the service that they are part of.

Ford and Honor identified that there are two groups of people that are potentially vulnerable to stress: younger inexperienced staff who were essentially undergoing a crisis of confidence and questioning their abilities as carers, and older, quite well-trained people who simply have 'run out of steam'.

Most organisations rely on the employment of significant numbers of casual workers, taking the form of staff supplied by an external agency or employed by the care providing organisation itself as a pool of staff for whom work is not guaranteed, but who can be drawn on in times of shortages. Sometimes such a pool of casual workers is referred to as the staff 'bank'.

Hardly anyone who participates in care work approves of the notion of casual workers. Permanent staff generally prefer to be supported by their regular colleagues whom they know well and are more likely to trust; bank or agency staff usually would rather have the guaranteed work, security and employment rights attached to a permanent job; service users may become distressed by the presence of unfamiliar casual staff and senior managers certainly resent the high cost of agency staff. Probably the only party that is satisfied by the need to use high levels of temporary staff consists of the proprietors of employment agencies whose profits benefit from an increased use of their workforce particularly during weekends, night time and bank holidays when premiums are higher.

Nevertheless, there may be very good reasons why temporary staff are used relating to deficiencies in the recruitment of regular team members, personal needs of casual workers and organisational reconfigurations necessitating a block on the employment of new staff until redeployment processes are completed. Casual staff can provide a degree of flexibility whilst often being a source of permanent workers in the future.

Casual workers are a fact of life and consist of a group of people who have very specific needs. Bank and agency staff frequently experience discriminatory approaches: they are not always welcomed by established teams and are readily stigmatised or blamed for failings in services. It is difficult for them to fully feel part of a team however much they work in a specific care setting. Because of their decreased opportunities to learn specific information about individuals, such as triggers, early signs of anger, and effective approaches to challenges, they are more likely to be the victims of service user aggression, an experience compounded by their limited access to all but the most basic training.

A radical, seemingly simplistic approach is to be very clear why there are high rates of bank and agency staff and do something to address why it is difficult to retain or recruit staff. Surprisingly, unless the employers receive extremely poor wages, the size of their salaries is not always as significant a factor of excessive staff attrition as you would think. Carers are astonishingly loyal to the people that they support, their colleagues and immediate managers. They value things like proximity of a service to where they themselves live, the stability provided by a familiar work environment and assurance that their shift requests will be respected and generally that they will be accorded respect.

Inadequate, uncaring and unsupportive leadership approaches are often at the heart of the reasons for people wanting to leave as are environments where people feel excessively scrutinised and mistrusted to do their job without being 'micro managed'.

The vast majority of people who undertake the care and support of people with learning disabilities have the interests of their clients entirely at heart and their good intentions mean that they usually welcome chances to demonstrate initiative and help people live a more fulfilled life and opportunities to develop themselves.

Morale amongst teams of carers can sometimes be a very delicate flower that can easily wilt in such adverse circumstances. Other factors which cause staff to lose heart and move on include feelings that they are not doing their job properly because they cannot provide an adequate lifestyle for the people that they support, being worn down by service users' challenges and characteristics, having to endure changes that they have little say in and regard as unnecessary and unhelpful. Sometimes they may have perceptions that their managers are remote, indifferent, uninspiring and unempathic.

Helen Sanderson (2003) talks of creating 'person-centred teams', comprising of people that are confident and assertive and who are given opportunities to act autonomously. Empowering staff members so that they can use their initiative and feel that they can make suggestions that will be respected and given full consideration is a way to counteract this trend. Of course, people can only take on more responsibility if they have received sufficient development so providing those learning opportunities help people to perform their roles better, increase their confidence and sense of self-worth and foster loyalty to their organisation.

Nevertheless, there will always be occasions when services do have to use temporary staff. How can the impact of those bank and agency workers be minimised for the benefit of both service users and staff morale?

It is good to create a dedicated team of staff who principally work in the one service, as their familiarity to clients and understanding of their needs is reassuring to service users and permanent staff alike. However, that is only possible if the substantive team is welcoming and helpful towards their temporary colleagues, rather than giving the impression that they regard the latter as inferior as and less capable than themselves. Casual workers must be made to feel that they are an intrinsic and valued part of the team to encourage them to return to a particular area. The support of people with learning disabilities is a very labour-intensive business and frequently casual workers can choose to avoid going to places where they feel devalued and unwelcome, because they know that there are many other opportunities elsewhere.

Other ways that bank workers can feel more valued and supported is through ensuring that they receive regular supervision sessions, easier said than achieved when someone habitually works in multiple settings, but possible when the bank worker has an allocated manager based at one of their regular venues who will take responsibility for ensuring that one to one sessions take place.

Each area needs to ensure that workplace induction for bank workers is started promptly and is detailed enough to guarantee that bank workers have sufficient knowledge to discharge their duties towards service users but are not overwhelmed by a surfeit of information. Regular staff have a part to play in matching the bank staff to particular clients and regulating the level of induction that is appropriate to supporting those individuals. Also, permanent staff need to check and support their temporary colleagues throughout their shifts and ensure that they are not asked to support individuals who have a level of complexity and need that is beyond the current abilities and experience of particular bank staff.

It is absolutely essential that bank and even agency staff are given all the necessary training that appertains to the client groups that they usually support. It is not uncommon for bank staff to have a preference for supporting service users with particular needs e.g. one person might like to care for elderly and frail people whilst others like to support profoundly physically and intellectually impaired individuals. Others prefer to work with people with complex emotional needs who may display problematic behaviours whilst some prefer to support very able people who are learning to live more independently. Each group requires quite a different skill set and different training needs and the more bank workers specialise in this manner the easier it is to deliver relevant training. It is only recently perhaps the appreciation of the need for casual staff to have the chance to formulate a Personal Development Plan with their supervisors and have access to training which is highly specific to their chosen client group and role.

Chapter 8
Stress, Burnout Organisational Factors
What do we mean by 'stress and burnout' and how is it experienced?

Stress can be considered to be a response to threat within an individual's environment when the demands placed upon them are greater than their personal resources for coping (Lazarus and Folkman, 1984).

Burnout, first described by Maslach and Jackson in 1981, is a phenomenon which can be experienced by those who work extensively with people, such as nurses, carers, social workers and teachers. It is a particular peril for members of those professions people who give a lot of emotional support or give more than they receive in return and is characterised by three elements: emotional exhaustion, depersonalisation, and reduced personal accomplishment (Thompson and Rose 2011). Translated into everyday language, carers may feel overwhelming wearied both physically and emotionally by their contact with disabled people; they may feel the need to become more emotionally detached from their clients, developing a sense of indifference and apathy or even cynicism; consequently they may form a perception of themselves as being less effective as carers than they used to be because their interactions with others are no longer lively and positive. Carers may become very guilty about this state of affairs and blame themselves for deterioration in service users' behaviours.

Devereux and others (2009) describe five models which attempt to explain how stress occurs in the workplace.

1)   The person-environment fit theory in which:

Stress does not arise from the work environment or due to individuals but is a result of a disparity of fit between environment and workers, a mismatch which causes strain associated with role demands that may be overwhelming, conflicting or ambiguous. This concept which is very reminiscent to that of 'Goodness of Fit' between service users and their environment postulated in Positive Behavioural Support literature as a desirable outcome for clients who challenge services.

2)   The demand – control model

This can be explained in two ways. The first perspective is demand-control-support (Karasek and Theorell 1990) in which stress arise from the dynamic between the carers' discernment of the demands and control that they encounter at work and the level of support that they think they are given. Secondly, the demands-control-constraints model (Payne 1979) asserts the significance of the tension between constraints, i.e. factors in the environment which impede carers' ability to meet demands, support that is given and the very demands of their job role.

3)   The cognitive-behavioural theory

This model suggests that stress arises from an initial appraisal of a situation ascertaining the degree of threat and a subsequent assessment of the person's ability to cope with and manage that situation.

4)   Emotional overload

Emotional overload relates to the demands experienced by carers during their interactions and relationships with clients. Demands can be quantitative, for example in the need to give continuous support, or qualitative as in the lack of effective support.

5) <u>Equity theory</u>

The assumption in this model of work stress is that we aspire to relationships which have a degree of equality and suffer distress if this is not so. In care and support settings roles are often circumscribed; carers are the active givers of support whilst the service user is a passive recipient, particularly if their intellectual capacities are extremely limited, leading to a lack of reciprocity and inequity within the relationship.

Devereaux and others (2009) remind us that stress is not inevitably harmful. Stress that is well managed can result in carers progressing and developing, a phenomenon sometimes termed term 'eustress', in contrast with circumstances where stress isn't well managed, has a negative effect and 'distress' occurs instead.

How do we know that carers are becoming stressed? We certainly can't rely on carers to necessarily report their negative feelings themselves. They may not have been intellectually equipped or temperamentally inclined to engage in an examination and disclosure of their emotions in such a conscious, self-analytical way. Also, they may believe that admitting to feeling stressed is a sign of weakness and would be interpreted by supervisors and managers as a sign of fallibility or even incompetence, possibly placing their employment in jeopardy.

There are several measures which are identified in the relevant research literature and are also regarded colloquially by people who work in the field as being significant, such as a high level of illness and absenteeism. This phenomenon is easily established as employers habitually keep detailed records about their employees' sick records, but with the primary intention to inform the need to use sanctions against members of the work to lower rates of absenteeism in order to ensure financial probity and preserve standards of care. As part of the process, people may be asked if there are any factors which are affecting their well-being and increasing their levels of stress. However, this is done in an incidental rather than systematic manner, with the focus understandably remaining on the needs of the service and ultimately those of service users.

Alternatively, carers may develop feelings of disaffection and alienation towards the parent organisation, which may manifest in a truculent, querulous, even intimidatory manner towards administrative and managerial staff, more likely to be interpreted as an attitudinal defect in those members of staff rather an indicator of a decrease in their morale.

Other indicators may be less immediate and very personal and so not readily ascertained. For instance, staff may seek to alleviate their distress by a form of self-medication, smoking cigarettes more frequently, drinking greater quantities of alcohol or consuming recreational drugs. They may develop eating disorders or disrupted sleep patterns and a decreased interest in their usual activities. They may experience a variety of psychiatric illnesses, such as anxiety and depression. Hatton and others (1999) established in their study that it is likely that one third of staff working in adult services for people with learning disabilities are likely to be so stressed that it is tantamount to having a mental health disorder, compared with 18% for the general population. Developing a physical illness is another possibility, such as stomach disorders, cardiovascular disease or 'type 2' diabetes, all of which are recognised as possible consequences of increased stress levels.

Sometimes there might be deterioration in the relationships that members of staff have with their colleagues and service users; they may be irritable towards the former or become withdrawn, whilst their interactions with clients are decreased both in quality and number, maybe culminating in abusive approaches. Occurrences of this nature inevitably and again understandably are dealt with as disciplinary issues when they do emerge. However, factors such as an increase in job strain might have contributed to carers following such a harmful route.

The literature appertaining to the stress experienced by carers who support people with learning disabilities make reference to several tools for either determining levels of stress and burnout or measuring staff attitudes to significant factors, such as challenging behaviour.

Maslach Burnout Inventory (Maslach and Jackson 1981; 1986)

This instrument, often abbreviated to MBI, is a 22-item survey that assesses professional burnout in caring occupations, human services, education, business and government professions principally in three areas, the first being 'Emotional Exhaustion': the experience of being emotionally overwhelmed and exhausted by your work. Secondly, it measures Depersonalisation: the sense of impersonal and apathetic feelings towards the clients for whom you are providing a service. Finally, MBI assesses 'Personal Accomplishment', how much you regard yourself as being competent at your work and your level of achievement. Developed by Dr Christine Maslach in 1981, MBI is regarded as a very credible and extensively validated instrument.

Thoughts and Feelings Index (Fletcher and Jones 1992)

This is a short questionnaire which measures the impact of job strain in various occupational groups and the resultant manifestation anxiety and depression. The Thoughts and Feelings Index is similar to the Crown-Crisp Experiential Index (Crown and Crisp 1979), which seeks to measure anxiety, obsessionality, depression, somatic anxiety, depression hysteria and phobic anxiety in a variety of contexts.

Malaise Stress Inventory (Rutter and others 1970)

This tool was developed originally as a means to assess stress experienced by the mothers of severely disabled children. The scale assesses symptoms related to twenty-four physical, emotional and psychosomatic items.

Occupational Stress Questionnaire or Job Stress Questionnaire (JSQ) (Caplan and others 1975)

This questionnaire includes the assessment of dimensions such as workload, role conflict, performance pressure, and role ambiguity.

Psychosocial Work Environment and Stress Questionnaire (Avergold 1998)

This scale examines the domains of job demands and control, workload, influence in decision making, management style, role clarity, social contact, both formal and informal contact with colleagues, social climate (cliques, conflicts and disagreements), personal development and work centrality, the importance of one's work and level of commitment to it. The questionnaire also contains scales to measure mental fatigue (including reluctance towards and reoccupation with work), psychological distress, such as irritability and depression, and psychosomatic symptoms like stomach or back pains, dizziness and palpitations. The amount of time spent on sick leave is also measured.

Occupational Stress Indicator or Inventory (Cooper and others 1988)

This measures areas, including sources of stress at work, individual factors or characteristics, coping strategies, and outcomes for both the individual and an organisation from employees suffering stress.

Staff Stressor Questionnaire (Hatton and others 1999)

Developed specifically to assess stressors for staff working with people who have learning disabilities, this seeks to assess the level of stress produced by seven factors: service user challenging behaviour, poor client skills, lack of staff support, lack of resources, the low-status of care work, bureaucracy and work-home conflict.

Social Support Questionnaire (Sarason and others 1983)

By the use of six key questions, this tool seeks to measure social supports and the number of available supportive individuals to which carers have access.

DASS 21 (Lovibond and Lovibond 1995)

This is a measure which assesses stress, anxiety and depression in members of a workforce that is regarded as suitable for use in healthcare or similar settings.

Survey of POS (Eisenberger and others 1990)

This tool is used to assess 'Perceived Organisational Support', the quantity and quality of support that workers believe that they receive from their managers and employers.

As can be seen there are many formats that could be used to assess the stress levels of the work force, all with slightly different perspectives, but united by the common condition that they are hardly ever used to assess the stress levels of carers unless as part of an academic study.

The impact of organisational/workplace issues

As might be expected, carers have a set of concerns relating to quite mundane but significant aspects of their working experience. The need to provide support usually over a 24-hour period and the resultant shift patterns leads to tensions around maintaining a reasonable balance between work and home life, meeting family demands and obligations, and pursuing a full social life. People find that the latter is particularly disrupted by weekend, late evening and night time working. If your friends predominantly have jobs which consist of working 9 to 5 from Monday to Friday, the impact of a shift pattern which entails working a high proportion of unsocial hours can be very noticeable and irksome.

Moreover, the requirement to work different types of shifts, sometimes combinations of 'earlies', 'lates' and 'nights' plus 'sleep-ins' (during which the member of staff remains at their workplace overnight, sleeping on the premises), within a relatively short time span produces physical and psychological strains not experienced by the vast majority of the population who follow more conventional working arrangements. People derive a great deal of emotional stability from the predictability of regular working patterns and practically it is easier for them to organise their personal lives around that set framework.

Working combinations of shifts, particularly if it periodically involves night duties and sleeping in, inevitably is tiring as it is difficult to establish a regular sleep pattern in these circumstances. Also 'nights' tend to be longer than the typical span of day shifts, whilst 'sleep-ins' often are sandwiched between late and early shifts. It is not unusual for a carer to start work at two thirty pm, finish at eleven pm, do a sleep-in until seven am the following day and then an early shift which finishes at one thirty pm a total span of twenty-three hours at the workplace. Of course, it is possible that the member of staff may be woken up during their 'sleep-in' either by ambient work place noise or because service users need their support for a variety of reasons. Shift patterns which entail such combinations, even if they are not as lengthy as the example that I have just cited, are always wearing especially if you are the only person on duty during that period.

A further potential disruption to carers' lives relates to the increasing tendency for spans of support to be related very closely to service users' needs and lead to an even more disjointed working week with little opportunity to establish a conventional sense of routine.

Organisations require staff to work shifts which are entirely consistent with the needs of service users. Therefore, carers might suddenly discover that they have to change individual shifts due to those needs with a consequent disruption of their personal lives and further erosion of the already limited sense of predictability that they have around working patterns.

Carers find it stressful when they have to work in situations where the staff complement is lower than usual, or the deficit is made up by the use of casual or agency staff.

With regards to the latter circumstance, regular staff experience a disproportionate burden of responsibility as they feel that they have to take the lead in organising care on those days.

This is because temporary staff may not necessarily have the knowledge and experience to take that lead themselves whereas usually that burden is shared with experienced and trusted colleagues who have a similar understanding of the very specific needs of their service users.

What can help to mitigate the impact of unsocial hours, an inevitable component of carers' working lives? Appointing managers should make it very clear to prospective employees the entire nature of the shift patterns that they would be working, including the precise hours, the likely mixture of shifts and quantity of weekend working emphasising that any unusual shift times, are not arbitrary but are devised to ensure that support is provided in a person centred way based on the needs and wishes of service users. Armed with this knowledge, they can make an informed decision as to whether care work of this nature is appropriate for them.

In residential settings, rotas should be constructed with great care ensuring that there is equity with respect to the allocation of the proportion of early, late and night shifts and that sleep-ins are also distributed fairly. Similarly, weekend duties should be allocated equally, unless, of course a member of staff has a preference for doing those shifts due to family circumstances. There may be a need to ask that staff occasionally fulfil unusual shift patterns due to the needs of service users, such as those appertaining to social activities and medical appointments. However, regimes which entail people doing 'split' shifts, where staff have a break of a few hours between periods of work a regular basis are likely to impact negatively on staff welfare.

Also, every effort must be made to ensure that there is a balance so that there are not a disproportionate number of inexperienced or temporary care workers on duty for any particular day.

Certainly, the main priority in compiling duty rotas is to ensure that the needs of service users are met. However, a request process for making requests should be in place, so that whoever is compiling the rota is aware of any particular individual need. Staff should have plenty of notice concerning their shift pattern and have opportunities to negotiate changes with colleagues as long as this is sanctioned by managers and does not affect service needs.

In smaller properties, sometimes the sleeping in arrangements are very Spartan, comprising a fold up bed in the lounge and limited privacy for the member of staff, plus, of course, a greater chance of being woken up because of the extreme proximity to the general living areas.

If there is a need for staff to do 'sleep-in' duties, a separate room, preferably with en-suite facilities, which offers suitable privacy, comfort and protection from ambient noise, should be provided. If sleeping in staff members are woken at night, they should routinely be given the option to go home early the following morning.

All of the above are simple, obvious and reasonable working conditions and approaches which should be adhered to uniformly by services in order to enhance staff well-being. Many organisations do so, but in times of financial constraint and decreased concern about employee welfare due to the incidence of high levels of unemployment, it easy to envisage that less concern could be given to these matters.

Weekend, evening and night time working affects the workforce in other ways. The disparity between the 9 to 5 weekday work patterns of administrative staff and senior managers compared to their own unsocial regime may be especially acutely felt when serious incidents occur during those hours, leaving staff feeling vulnerable and isolated.

Sometimes a simple expedient, such as home and project managers occasionally doing shifts and working at weekends, can be a help. Team members feel that the manager is demonstrating solidarity with their staff, a resolve to learn about situations that develop during weekends and evenings and a willingness to provide support at those times.

When asked, team members generally have very clear ideas concerning what they prefer in terms of support and approach from an organisation. They like to know that they are respected as individuals, that their contributions are valued, that they are given some degree of autonomy and opportunities to display initiative. However, they like to know that they will be supported if they are involved in situations which are controversial or beyond their level of responsibility and skill or training level.

Rightfully, organisations which provide care and support for the most vulnerable groups in society such as the elderly, those who have enduring mental ill health and people with learning disabilities have much higher standards and expectations nowadays. As a result, investigations relating to conduct by carers are probably more frequent. It is vital that all suspicions of impropriety are investigated to the fullest extent particularly in circumstances when abuse against service users is alleged.

Nevertheless, although the 'garden leave' (a period of time where the person is asked to stay away from work until a formal decision is made as to the best way forward) or suspension that is usually imposed whilst an investigation is pursued is not meant to imply that the subject of investigation is culpable, in practice stigma and an assumption of malpractice is often assumed when staff do undergo this process. It is inevitable that members of staff who undergo enforced leave of this nature are going to feel very isolated and vulnerable. They will have plenty of free time on their hands to dwell on their predicament and because they are obliged to refrain from contact with their workplace, they are denied the usual support from their colleagues.

What is helpful to staff who are going through this process, irrespective of their level of culpability, is ongoing and frequent support from a nominated colleague, whether a senior manager or Human Resources adviser.

Final Thoughts

To the best of my knowledge no-one has ever written a whole book on the support needs of professional carers who work with people who have learning disabilities. There have been plenty of specialist journal articles which inevitably have a limited readership, confined to people who work in the academic field.

For many there may be little justification for such a lengthy piece of work, especially as often carers do not recognise or dismissive of the factors that I have identified and discussed in the previous chapters.

However, those factors, many identified through research, and the formulation of strategies to address them remain very necessary for many reasons.

It makes good business sense to look after staff, they are less likely to become ill and cause added costs by having lengthy or frequent periods of sickness; they are more likely to remain in post again avoiding the disruption and expense of more recruitment. There is a legal obligation to pay attention to the welfare of carers driven by the need to conform to Health and Safety law. Employers have a moral imperative to care for staff; this seems particularly apposite when the purpose of an organisation is to provide care to disadvantaged groups of people. Finally, service users themselves are going to be the greatest beneficiaries of a more considered and sophisticated approach to staff support needs which ensures that carers' stress levels and working conditions are minimised.

The necessity to make progress in these areas seems incontestable, the existence of the will and energy to do so remains doubtful…

Bibliography

Avergold, M. 1998: *The Psychosocial Work Environment and Stress Questionnaire* (PWESQ). Copenhagen: The Danish Work Environment Fund.

Belbin, RM. 2010: *Team Roles at Work*. London: Butterworth-Heinemann.

Breakwell, GM. 1997: *Coping with Aggressive Behaviour*. Leicester: British Psychological Society.

Briggs Myers, I. 2000: *An Introduction to Type: A Guide to Understanding Your Results on the Myers-Briggs Type Indicator*. Oxford: Oxford Psychologists Press.

Bromley, J and Emerson, E. 1995: "Beliefs and emotional reactions of care staff working with people with challenging behaviour." *Journal of Intellectual Disability Research*, 39(4), pp. 341-52

Caplan, RD; Cobb, S; French, JR; Van Harrison, R; and Pinneau Jr, SR. 1975: *Job Demands and Worker Health: Main Effects and Occupational Differences*. Ann Arbor: US Dept. of Health and Welfare.

Cooper, L and Bright, J. 2001: "Individual differences in reactions to stress." Jones, F and Bright, J (Eds), *Stress: Myth, theory and research.* Harlow, England: Pearson Education.

Crown, S and Crisp, AH. 1979: *Manual of the Crown-Crisp Experiential Index*. London: Hodder and Stoughton.

Cudré-Mauroux, A. 2009: "Staff attributions about challenging behaviours of people with intellectual disabilities and transactional stress process: A qualitative study." *Journal of Intellectual Disability Research*, 54(1), pp. 26-39.

Cudré-Mauroux, A. 2011: "Self-efficacy and stress of staff managing challenging behaviours of people with learning disabilities." *British Journal of Learning Disabilities*, 39(3), pp. 181-89.

Devereux, J; Hastings, R; and Noone, S. 2009: "Staff stress and burnout in intellectual disability services: Work stress theory and its application." *Journal of Applied Research in Intellectual Disabilities*, 22(6), pp. 561–73.

Duran, A; Extremera, N; and Rey, L. 2004: "Self-reported emotional intelligence, burnout and engagement among staff in services for people with intellectual disabilities." *Psychological Reports*, 95(2), pp. 386-90.

Dyer, L and Quine, L. 1998: "Predictors of job satisfaction and burnout among the direct care staff of a community learning disability service." *Journal of Applied Research In Intellectual Disabilities*, 11(4), pp. 320-32.

Eisenburger, R; Fasolo, P; and Davis-LaMastro, V. 1990: "Perceived organisational support and employee diligence, commitment, and innovation." *Journal of Applied Psychology*, 75(1), pp. 51-59.

Elliott, JL and Rose, J. 1997: "An investigation of stress experienced by managers of community homes for people with intellectual disabilities." *Journal of Applied Research in Intellectual Disabilities*, 10(1), pp. 48-53.

Fletcher, BC and Jones, F. 1992: "Measuring Organizational Culture: The Cultural Audit." *Managerial Auditing Journal*, 7(6), pp. 30-36.

Ford, J and Honnor, J. 2000: "Job satisfaction of community residential staff serving individuals with severe intellectual disabilities." *Journal of Intellectual and Developmental Disability*, 25(4), pp. 343-62.

Gardner, B; Rose, J; Mason, O; Tyler, P; and Cushway, D. 2005: "Cognitive therapy and behavioural coping in the management of work-related stress: An intervention study." *Work & Stress: An International Journal of Work, Health, & Organisations*, 19(2), pp. 137-52.

Harris, P and Rose, J. 2002: "Measuring staff support in services for people with intellectual disability: The Staff Support and Satisfaction Questionnaire, Version 2." *Journal of Intellectual Disability Research*, 46(2), pp. 151-57.

Hastings, RP. 2002: "Do challenging behaviours affect staff psychological well-being? Issues of causality and mechanism." *American Journal on Mental Retardation*, 107(6), pp. 455-67.

Hastings, RP and Brown, T. 2002: "Coping strategies and the impact of challenging behaviours on special educators' burnout." *Mental Retardation*, 40(2), pp.148-56.

Hastings, RP and Horne, S. 2004: "Positive perceptions held by support staff in community mental retardation services." *American Journal on Mental Retardation*, 109(1), pp.53-62.

Hastings, RP; Horne, S; and Mitchell, G. 2004: "Burnout in direct care staff in intellectual disability services: a factor analytical study of the Maslach Burnout Inventory." *Journal of Intellectual Disability Research*, 48(3), pp. 268-73.

Hatton, C; Brown, R; Caine, A; and Emerson, E. 1995: "Stressors, coping strategies and stress-related outcomes among direct care staff in staffed houses for people with learning disabilities." *Mental Handicap Research*, 8(4), pp. 252-71.

Hatton, C; Emerson, E; Rivers, M; Mason, H; Mason, L; Swarbrick, R; Kiernan, C; Reeves, D; and Alborz, A. 1999: "Factors associated with staff stress and work satisfaction in services for people with intellectual disability." *Journal of Intellectual Disability Research*, 43(4), pp. 253-67.

Hatton, C; Rivers, M; Mason, H; Mason, L; Emerson, E; Kiernan, C; Reeves, D; and Alborz, A. 1999: "Organisational culture and staff outcomes in services for people with intellectual disabilities." *Journal of Intellectual Disability Research*, 43(3), pp. 206-18.

Hatton, C; Rivers, M; Mason, H; Mason, L; Kiernan, C; Emerson, E; Alborz, A; and Reeves, D. 1999: "Staff stressors and staff outcomes in services for adults with intellectual disabilities: The Staff Stressor Questionnaire." *Research in Developmental Disabilities*, 20(4), pp. 269-85.

Hatton, C; Emerson, E; Rivers, M; Mason, H; Mason, L; Swarbrick, R; Kiernan, C; Reeves, D; and Alborz, A. 2001: "Factors associated with intended staff turnover and job search behaviour in services for people with intellectual disability." *Journal of Intellectual Disability Research*, 45(3), pp. 258-70.

Hill, C and Dagnan, D. 2002: "Helping, attributions, emotions and coping style in response to people with learning disabilities and challenging behaviour." *Journal of Learning Disabilities*, 6(4), pp. 363-72.

Honey, P and Mumford, A. 1989: *The Manual of Learning Opportunities*. Peter Honey Publications.

Innstrand, ST; Espnes, GA; and Mykletum, R. 2004: "Job stress, burnout and job satisfaction: An intervention study for staff working with people with intellectual disabilities." *Journal of Applied Research in Intellectual Disabilities*, 17(2), pp. 119-26.

Jenkins, R; Rose, J; and Lovell, C. 1998: "Psychological well-being of staff working with people who have challenging behaviour." *Journal of Intellectual Disability Research*, 41(6), pp. 502-11.

Karasek, RA and Theorell, T. 1990: *Healthy Work: Stress, Productivity, and the Reconstruction of Working Life*. New York: Basic Books.

Kobasa, SC; Maddi, SR; and Kahn, S. 1982: "Hardiness and health: A prospective study." *Journal of Personality and Social Psychology*, 42(1), pp. 168-77.

Lazarus, RS and Folkman, S. 1984: *Stress, Appraisal, and Coping*. New York: Spring Pub. Co.

Lernihan, E and Sweeney, J. 2010: "Measuring levels of burnout among care workers." *Learning Disability Practice*, 13(8), p 27-33.

Loehr, JE. 1995: *The New Toughness Training for Sports: Mental, Emotional, and Physical Conditioning from One of the World's Premier Sports Psychologists*. London: Plume.

Lovibond, PF and Lovibond, SH. 1995: "The structure of negative emotional states: Comparison of the Depression Anxiety Stress Scales (DASS) with the Beck Depression and Anxiety Inventories." *Behaviour Research and Therapy*, 33(3), pp. 335-43.

Lundström, M; Graneheim, UH; Eisemann, M; Richter, J; and Åström, S. 2005: "Influence of work climate for experiences of strain." *Learning Disability Practice*, 8(10), pp. 32-38.

MacGregor, D. 1960: *The Human Side of Enterprise*. New York: McGraw-Hill Book Co.

Maslach, C and Jackson, SE. 1986: *Maslach Burnout Inventory (2nd Edition)*. Palo Alto, CA: Consulting Psychologists Press.

Maslach, C; Jackson, S; Leiter, M. 1996: *Maslach Burnout Inventory Manual*. Palo Alto, CA: Consulting Psychologists Press.

Mitchell, G and Hastings, RP. 2001: "Coping, burnout, and emotion in staff working in community services for people with challenging behaviours." *American Journal on Mental Retardation*, 106(5), pp. 448-59.

McCallion, P; McCarron, M; and Force, LT. 2005: "A measure of subjective burden for dementia care: The Caregiving Difficulty Scale-Intellectual Disability." *Journal of Intellectual Disability Research*, 49(5), pp. 365-71.

McCarron, M and McCallion, P. 2005: "A revised stress and coping framework for staff carers of persons with intellectual disabilities and dementia." *Journal of Policy and Practice in Intellectual Disabilities*, 2(2), pp. 139-48.

Murray, GC; Sinclair, B; Kidd, GR; Quigley, A and McKenzie, K. 1999: "The relationship between staff sickness levels and client assault levels in a health service unit for people with an intellectual disability and severely challenging behaviour." *Journal of Applied Research in Intellectual Disabilities*, 12(3), pp. 263-68.

Mutkins, E; Brown, RF; and Thorsteinsson, EB. 2011: "Stress, depression. workplace and social supports and burnout in intellectual disability support staff." *Journal of Intellectual Disability Research*, 55(5) pp. 500-10.

Noone, SJ and Hastings, RP. 2009: "Building psychological resilience in support staff caring for people with intellectual disabilities Pilot evaluation of an acceptance-based intervention." *Journal of Intellectual Disabilities*, 13(1), pp. 43-53.

O'Brien, CL and O'Brien, J. 2002: "The origins of person-centred planning." O'Brien, J and O'Brien, CL (Eds), *Implementing Person-Centred Planning: Voices of Experience*, Vol. II. Toronto: Inclusion Press.

Paterson, B; Wilkinson, D; Leadbetter, D; Bradley, P; Bowie, V; and Martin, A. 2001: "How corrupted cultures lead to abuse of restraint interventions." *Learning Disability Practice*, 14(7), pp. 24-28.

Payne, RL. 1979: "Demands, supports, constraints and psychological health." Mackay, CJ and Cox, T (Eds), *Response to stress: Occupational aspects*. London: International Pub. Corp.

Raczka, R. 2005: "A focus group enquiry into stress experienced by staff working with people with challenging behaviours." *Journal of Intellectual Disabilities*, 9(2), pp. 167-77.

Rose, D and Rose, J. 2005: "Staff in services for people with intellectual disabilities: The impact of stress on attributions of challenging behaviour." *Journal of Intellectual Disability Research*, 49(11), pp. 827-38.

Rose, J. 1993: "Stress and staff in residential settings: The move from hospital to the community." *Mental Handicap Research*, 6(4), pp. 312-32.

Rose, J. 1995: "Stress and residential staff: Towards an integration of existing research." *Mental Handicap Research*, 8(4), pp. 220-36.

Rose, J. 1999: "Stress and residential staff who work with people who have an intellectual disability: A factor analytical study." *Journal of Intellectual Disability Research*, 43(4), pp. 268-78.

Rose, JL and Cleary, A. 2007: "Care staff perceptions of challenging behaviour and fear of assault." *Journal of Intellectual and Developmental Disability*, 32(2), pp.153-61.

Rose, J; David, G; and Jones, C. 2003: "Staff who work with people who have intellectual disabilities: The importance of personality." *Journal of Applied Research in Intellectual Disabilities*, 16(4), pp. 267-77.

Rose, J; Jones, C; and Elliott, JL. 2000: "Differences in stress levels between managers and direct care staff in group homes." *Journal of Applied Intellectual Disabilities*, 13(4), pp. 276-82.

Rose, J; Jones, F; and Fletcher, BC. 1998: "Investigating the relationship between stress and worker behaviour." *Journal of Intellectual Disability Research*, 42(2), pp. 163-72.

Rose, J; Jones, F; and Fletcher, BC. 1998: "The impact of a stress management programme on staff well-being and performance at work." *Work & Stress: An International Journal of Work, Health, & Organisations*, 12(2), pp. 112-24.

Rose, J; Ahuja, AK; and Jones, C. 2006: "Attitudes of direct care staff towards external professionals, team climate and psychological wellbeing: A pilot study." *Journal of Intellectual Disabilities*, 10(2), pp.105-20.

Rose, J and Schelewa-Davies, D. 1997: "The relationship between staff stress and team climate in residential services." *Journal of Learning Disabilities for Nursing, Health and Social Care*, 1(1), pp. 19-24.

Rutter, M; Tizard, J; and Whitmore, K. 1970: *Education, Health and Behaviour*. London: Longmans.

Sanderson, H. 2003: "Implementing person-centred planning by developing person-centred teams." *International Journal of Integrated Care*, 11(3), pp. 18-25.

Sanderson, H; Kennedy, J; Ritchie, P; with Goodwin, G. 1997: *People Plans and Possibilities: Exploring Person Centred Planning*. Edinburgh: SHS Trust.

Sandhu, DK; Rose, J; Rostill-Brookes, HJ; Thrift, S. 2012: "'It's intense, to an extent': A qualitative study of the emotional challenges faced by staff working on a treatment programme for intellectually disabled sex offenders." *Journal of Applied Research in Intellectual Disabilities*, 25(4), pp. 308-18.

Sarason, IG; Levine, HM; Basham, RB; and Sarason, BR. 1983: "Assessing social support: The Social Support Questionnaire." *Journal of Personality and Social Psychology*, 44(1), pp. 127-39.

Skirrow, P and Hatton, C. 2006: "'Burnout' amongst direct care workers in services for adults with learning disabilities: A systematic review of research findings and initial normative data." *Journal of Applied Research in Intellectual Disabilities*, 20(2), pp. 131-44.

Shaddock, AJ; Hill, M; and van Limbeek, CAH. 1998: "Factors associated with burnout in workers in residential facilities for people with an intellectual disability." *Journal of Intellectual and Developmental Disability*, 23(4), pp. 309-18.

Sharrard, HE. 1992: "Feeling the strain: Job stress and satisfaction of direct-care staff in the mental handicap service." *British Journal of Mental Subnormality*, 38(74), pp. 32-38.

Strand, ML; Benzein, E; and Saveman, BI. 2004: "Violence in the care of adult persons with intellectual disabilities." *Journal of Clinical Nursing*, 13(4), pp. 506-14.

Tredgold, AF. 1908: *Mental Deficiency (Amentia)*. London: Baillière & Co.

Wardhaugh, J and Wilding, P. 1998: "Towards an explanation of the corruption of care." Allott, M and Robb, M (Eds), *Understanding Health and Social Care: An Introductory Reader*. London: SAGE in association with The Open University.

CPSIA information can be obtained
at www.ICGtesting.com
Printed in the USA
LVHW082101110123
736979LV00009B/228

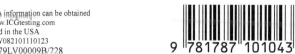